Practical Veterinary
Diagnostic Imaging

Companion website

This book is accompanied by a companion website:

www.wiley.com/go/easton/diagnosticimaging

The website includes:

- Case studies
- All figures as powerpoint slides
- Additional anatomy X-rays
- Guideline answers to the end-of-chapter Revision Questions found in the book

Practical Veterinary Diagnostic Imaging

Second Edition

Suzanne Easton

MSc, BSc (Hons), PGCertEd
*Senior Lecturer, Faculty of Health and Life Sciences,
University of West of England, Bristol*

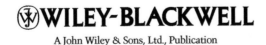

A John Wiley & Sons, Ltd., Publication

This edition first published 2012
© 2002 by Reed Educational and Professional Publishing Ltd
© 2012 by John Wiley & Sons Ltd

Wiley-Blackwell is an imprint of John Wiley & Sons, formed by the merger of Wiley's global Scientific, Technical and Medical business with Blackwell Publishing.

Registered office: John Wiley & Sons, Ltd, The Atrium, Southern Gate, Chichester, West Sussex, PO19 8SQ, UK

Editorial offices: 9600 Garsington Road, Oxford, OX4 2DQ, UK
The Atrium, Southern Gate, Chichester, West Sussex, PO19 8SQ, UK
2121 State Avenue, Ames, Iowa 50014-8300, USA

First published 2002
Second edition 2012

For details of our global editorial offices, for customer services and for information about how to apply for permission to reuse the copyright material in this book please see our website at www.wiley.com/wiley-blackwell.

The right of the author to be identified as the author of this work has been asserted in accordance with the UK Copyright, Designs and Patents Act 1988.

Library of Congress Cataloging-in-Publication Data
Easton, Suzanne.
  Practical veterinary diagnostic imaging / Suzanne Easton. – 2nd ed.
    p. ; cm.
  Rev. ed. of: Practical radiography for veterinary nurses / Suzanne Easton. 2002.
  Includes bibliographical references and index.
  ISBN 978-0-470-65648-8 (pbk. : alk. paper)   1. Veterinary radiography.
2. Veterinary diagnostic imaging. I. Easton, Suzanne. Practical radiography for veterinary nurses. II. Title.
  [DNLM: 1. Radiography–veterinary. SF 757.8]
  SF757.8.E38 2012
  636.089′607572–dc23

                                                                    2012010602

A catalogue record for this book is available from the British Library.

Wiley also publishes its books in a variety of electronic formats. Some content that appears in print may not be available in electronic books.

Cover image: iStockphoto.com
Cover design by Steve Thompson

Set in 10/12.5pt Plantin by Aptara® Inc., New Delhi, India

1   2012

Contents

Figure Acknowledgements   xi

1   Essential Mathematics and Physics   **1**
Matter, energy, power and heat   1
Units and prefixes used in radiography   3
Radiological units   4
Useful mathematics   7
Proportions and the inverse square law   7

2   The Principles of Physics Used in Radiography   **11**
Electrostatics – the electric charge   12
Conductors and insulators   14
Electricity   14
Measuring electricity   14
Types of current   15
Laws of an electric current   16
Resistance   16
Making a circuit – the options   17
Magnetism   17
The function and composition of a magnet   19
Magnetic laws   20
Electromagnetism – electricity and magnetism in union   21
Laws of electromagnetic induction   22
Further reading   23

3   Inside the Atom   **25**
Atoms, elements and other definitions   26
The 'Make-Up' of an atom – atomic structure   27
Shells and energy   28
The periodic table   28
Radioactivity   30
The effects of an electron changing orbits   30
Electromagnetic radiation   31

Frequency and wavelength   32
Further reading   33

4   **The X-ray Tube**   **35**
The tube housing   37
The cathode   39
The anode   42
The line focus principle   44
The anode-heel effect   45
The stator assembly   45
Tube rating   46
How to look after your X-ray tube   47
Further reading   47

5   **Diagnostic Equipment**   **49**
The X-ray circuit   50
What is seen from the outside?   51
High-voltage generators   51
Rectification   51
Mains supply switch   52
Primary circuit   52
Operating console   53
Filament circuit – control of the mA   54
High-tension circuit – provision of kV   55
Making an exposure – switches, timers and interlocks   55
Types of X-ray machines   56
Health and safety requirements   59
Power rating   59
Further reading   59

6   **Production of X-rays**   **61**
Electron production   62
Target interactions   63
X-ray emission spectrum   64
Altering the emission spectrum   65
X-ray quantity   68
X-ray quality   68
Altering exposure factors   68
Exposure charts   70
Further reading   70

7   **The Effects of Radiation**   **71**
The effect of the X-ray beam striking another atom   72
Absorption   75
Attenuation   75

The effects of ionising radiation on the body   76
Luminescence   77
Further reading   78

8 Control of the Primary Beam and Scatter   79
Light beam diaphragm   80
Factors affecting scattered radiation   81
Function of grids   81
Construction of a grid   82
Types of grid   84
Choosing a grid   85
Problems with using a grid   85
Air gap technique   86
Further reading   86

9 Radiographic Film   89
Film construction   90
Types of film   93
Formation of the latent image   94
Care and storage of films   95
Film sensitivity   96
Further reading   98

10 Intensifying Screens and Cassettes   99
The construction of intensifying screens   100
Film–screen combinations   101
Film–screen contact   104
Care of intensifying screens   104
Construction of cassettes   105
Care and use of cassettes   106
Further reading   106

11 Processing the Radiographic Film   107
The stages of processing   108
Developer   111
Fixer   112
Parts of the automatic processor   114
Replenishment   116
Silver recovery   117
The darkroom   118
Control of substances hazardous to health (COSHH)
  regulations   121
Other methods of processing   121
Further reading   122

12 Digital Radiography   **125**
Computed radiography   127
Care of the imaging plate and cassette   129
Computerised radiography process   129
Digital radiography   131
Image storage   133
Image display   134
Image quality   135
Further reading   135

13 Radiographic Image Quality   **137**
Sensitometry   138
Densitometry   138
Characteristic curve   139
Latitude   140
Density   141
Contrast   141
Magnification   144
Distortion   144
Movement   145
Producing a high-quality radiograph   146
Commonly seen film faults   147
Further reading   152

14 Radiation Protection   **153**
The effects of ionising radiation on the body   154
The basics to remember   154
Ionising Radiation Regulations 1999   155
Radiation safety in the veterinary practice   155
Classifying the areas around an X-ray machine   156
Dose limits   157
Monitoring devices   158
Lead shielding   159
Quality assurance   160
Further reading   161

15 Radiography Principles   **163**
General principles   164
Restraint   164
Positioning aids   165
Markers and legends   165
Assessing the radiograph   166
Terminology   166
BVA/KC hip dysplasia and elbow scoring scheme   168
Further reading   169

16 Contrast Media   **171**
     Negative contrast medium   172
     Positive contrast medium   172
     Contrast examination procedures   175
     Myelography   182
     Other contrast examinations   184
     Further reading   186

17 Small Animal Radiography Techniques   **189**
     Chest   189
     Abdomen   191
     Head and neck   192
     Distal extremities   196
     Shoulder   198
     Pelvis   200
     Spine   201
     Small mammals   202
     Birds   203
     Reptiles   204

18 Large Animal Radiography Techniques   **205**
     Foot   205
     Fetlock   207
     Metacarpus and metatarsus (cannon and splint)   209
     Carpus   209
     Elbow   211
     Shoulder   212
     Tarsus   213
     Stifle   214
     Head   216
     Spine   216
     Chest   217

19 Introduction to Ultrasound   **219**
     Sound waves   220
     Ultrasound   220
     How ultrasound works   220
     Types of ultrasound scan   222
     Doppler ultrasound   223
     Effects on tissue   224
     Ultrasound machines and transducers   224
     Patient preparation   225
     Areas suitable for examination   225
     Further reading   226

20   Advance Imaging Techniques   **227**
      Fluoroscopy   228
      Computerised tomography (CT)   230
      Magnetic resonance imaging (MRI)   232
      Nuclear scintigraphy   234
      Further reading   238

Index   239

Companion website

This book is accompanied by a companion website:

www.wiley.com/go/easton/diagnosticimaging

The website includes:

- Case studies
- All figures as powerpoint slides
- Additional anatomy X-rays
- Guideline answers to the end-of-chapter Revision Questions found in the book

Figure Acknowledgements

Figures 3.1, 3.4, 4.1, 7.3, 15.1 and 19.7
Aspinall, V. (2010) *Complete Textbook of Veterinary Nursing*, 2nd edn. Oxford: Elsevier.

Figures 4.4, 4.5 and 4.6
Bushong, S.C. (2004) *Radiological Science for Technologies: Physics, Biology and Protection*, 8th edn. St Louis: Mosby.

Figures 4.3, 6.6, 6.7, 6.8 and 8.1
Carter, P. (2007) *Imaging Science*. Oxford: Wiley-Blackwell.

Figures 5.5, 9.3, 9.5, 10.2, 12.2, 12.3, 12.4, 12.5, 12.6, 12.7, 12.8, 12.9 and 13.2
Easton, S. (2010) *An Introduction to Radiography*. Oxford: Churchill Livingstone.

Figures 1.1, 4.2, 4.8, 8.2, 8.3, 8.4, 8.5, 9.1, 9.2, 9.4, 11.2, 11.5, 12.1, 13.1, 13.5 and 13.6
Fauber, T. (2004) *Radiographic Imaging and Exposure*, 2nd edn. St Louis: Mosby.

Figures 2.7, 4.7 and 10.1
Graham, D., Cloke, P., Vosper, M. (2007) *Principles of Radiological Physics*, 5th edn. Edinburgh: Churchill Livingstone.

Figures 18.3, 18.4, 18.5, 18.6, 18.8 and 18.9
Han, C., Hurd, C. (2005) *Practical Diagnostic Imaging for the Veterinary Technician*, 3rd edn. St Louis: Mosby.

Figures 17.3, 17.4, 17.6, 17.7, 17.9, 17.10, 17.12, 17.14 and 17.15
Lavin, L. (2007) *Radiography in Veterinary Technology*, 4th edn. St Louis: Mosby.

Figures 18.1, 18.2, 18.7, 18.10 and 18.11
Mendenhall, A., Cantwell, H.D. (1988) *Equine Radiographic Procedures*. Philadelphia: Lea and Febiger.

Figures 3.3, 6.3, 6.4, 7.1, 7.2 and 15.2
Thrall, D. (2002) *Textbook of Veterinary Diagnostic Radiology*, 4th edn. Philadelphia: W.B. Saunders.

Figures 19.1, 20.3, 20.6 and 20.9
Patel, P.R. (1997) *Lecture Notes on Radiology*. Oxford: Blackwell Science.

Figures 5.1, 5.3 and 5.4
Xograph Healthcare Ltd. and Cave Veterinary Specialists.

Chapter 1

Essential Mathematics and Physics

Chapter contents

Matter, energy, power and heat
Units and prefixes used in radiography
Radiological units
Useful mathematics
Proportions and the inverse square law

Introduction

This chapter introduces and explores the principles of mathematics
and physics that will make following chapters and the principles of
radiography easier to understand. Although many of the concepts
introduced in this chapter are only for revision, they are relevant to
later chapters.

Matter, energy, power and heat

Matter

The entire world is made up of matter. Anything that occupies space
can be termed 'matter'. Matter is a collection of atoms, the basic
building blocks. All matter has mass, that is, the measure of matter
in an actual object. If gravity is involved, this mass is known as the
weight of an object. If an object is placed in a lesser gravitational field,
such as the atmosphere on the moon, the mass will remain the same,
but the weight will decrease. The weight will also change if the object
changes form, but, again, the mass will remain the same. An example
of this is water in its three forms – solid (ice), liquid (water) and gas
(steam). In these three forms, the mass is the same throughout, but
the weight changes considerably.

Matter	**A collection of atoms and molecules**
Mass	**The measure of matter in an object**
Weight	**Mass under the influence of gravity**

Practical Veterinary Diagnostic Imaging, Second Edition. Suzanne Easton.
© 2012 John Wiley & Sons, Ltd. Published 2012 by Blackwell Publishing Ltd.

Energy

The process of matter altering its state or form produces energy. Any object, however large or small, that is able to do 'work' is said to have energy. Energy has a number of different forms. Energy can be neither created nor destroyed, although it can change from one form to another (Table 1.1).

> **Total energy is measured in joules (J):**
>
> **Total energy = Potential energy + Kinetic energy**

Table 1.1   Energy types, definitions and examples.

Energy type	Description	Example
Potential	The amount of work an object could do because of its position	An axe raised, ready to be brought down to chop, has potential energy
Kinetic	As an object leaves its state of potential energy, it gains kinetic energy	An apple gains kinetic energy as it falls out of a tree
Electrical	The movement of electrons inside a conductor after the application of a potential difference	The movement of electrons in a cable produces the electrical energy needed to make a bulb light up
Nuclear	Nuclear energy is the energy stored within the nucleus of an atom	This energy is formed when the nucleus of an atom is split
Thermal	The energy of a hot object. This is caused by the vibration of molecules within matter	A hot bath has faster moving molecules than a cool bath
Sound	The energy produced by sound vibrations	A musical instrument, engine noise, speech, thunder, diagnostic ultrasound, sonar
Chemical	The energy generated when a reaction occurs between two substances	Thermal energy produced when water is added to hot oil
Electromagnetic	Electric and magnetic energy moving in waves	X-ray production, radio waves, infrared light

Energy conversion

As energy cannot be created or destroyed, it changes form, and this process is known as energy conversion.

In radiography, the X-ray tube is an example where energy is converted from one form (electrical) into other forms (X-rays, heat, light). We also use ultrasound where an ultrasound transducer converts electrical energy into sound energy, and the reflected sound energy is converted back into electrical energy.

Power

Power is the rate of doing work or the rate of transforming energy. This is measured in joules per second or watts. In radiography, due to the amount of energy transformation occurring, power is measured in thousands of watts or kilowatts (kW). A typical X-ray room will have a 50-kW generator to supply electric power to the X-ray equipment.

> **Power is measured in joules per second (J s⁻¹) or watts (W).**

Heat

Heat is the total energy of atoms and molecules moving in matter. The average speed of movement is known as temperature. Heat always flows from hot to cold until an equilibrium is reached. This movement can occur through three different methods – convection, conduction and radiation (Table 1.2). The rate of heat loss or transfer will depend on the type of surface material and the difference between the two areas of heat. This is utilised in an X-ray tube through the choice of material used for the anode and the colour of the tube head (black).

Table 1.2 Definitions of conduction, convection and radiation.

Convection	This occurs in liquids and gases. The matter moves, taking the heat with it. This occurs because of the reduction in density associated with heating. Hotter material rises and displaces cooler material above. This is the principle behind surrounding an X-ray tube in oil as a cooling technique.
Conduction	This is found in metals. The heat is transferred through contact, with heat flowing from the hot area to the cooler area. This principle is used in the anode and stem of the X-ray tube.
Radiation	Vibrating molecules on the surface of matter generate electromagnetic waves. Energy in the form of heat leaves the surface and transfers the energy to whatever it strikes. This is most effective in a vacuum.

Units and prefixes used in radiography

The use of scientific terminology in radiography is based on standardised units and prefixes to abbreviate large or very small numbers. It also provides an international language amongst radiographers. The use of standardised units extends to the description of units of measure and the identification of units of ionising radiation.

Standard scientific notation

Radiography uses both very large units and very small units. Examples of this are the 100,000 volts necessary to radiograph a chest and the 0.004 amperes (amps) needed to demonstrate a cat's carpus. These are two of the core units used in radiography and are described as kilovolts (kV) and milliamperes (mA). Using this notation, 100,000 volts is described as 100 kV and 0.004 amperes as 4 mA. Where large numbers are used, the numbers can also be described as exponents. Exponents describe numbers as multiples of ten (the system most widely used in everyday life is the decimal system; see Table 1.3).

Table 1.3 Standard scientific notation, prefixes and symbols.

Notation	Decimal number	Prefix	Symbol
10^9	1,000,000,000	giga-	G
10^6	1,000,000	mega-	M
10^3	1000	kilo-	k
10^2	100	hecto-	h
10^1	10	deka-	da
10^{-1}	0.1	deci-	d
10^{-2}	0.01	centi-	c
10^{-3}	0.001	milli-	m
10^{-6}	0.000001	micro-	μ

SI base units

In order to maintain a common radiographic language, the units used as a baseline for measurements and discussions need to be standardised. Radiography uses the International System of Units or 'SI'. Problems would occur if the focus-to-film distance was given in metres on the practice exposure chart and the veterinary nurse carrying out examinations worked in inches. The base units in Table 1.4 are the units used to calculate more complicated measures such as speed (m s^{-1}) or force (kg m s^{-2}). There are seven base units from which all other units are derived.

Radiological units

Radiology has a number of units specific to the field that are in common use (see Table 1.5). These are all related to the measurement of the production of X-rays and the effect of the energy produced, and

Table 1.4 SI units used in radiography.

Term	SI unit	Definition	Application to radiography
Energy	Joule J	Ability to do work	Production of X-rays
Mass	Kilogram kg	A measure of the number of atoms and molecules in a body	Important when determining the radiation dose to a patient
Gray	Joules per kilogram Gy	Energy imparted to a body by ionising radiation	Unit of radiation dose measurement
Power	Joules per second W	Rate of doing work	Output of X-ray generator
Electric current	Ampere A	Movement of electrons flowing per unit time	Quantity of electrons flowing per unit time
Electric charge	Coulomb C	One ampere flowing per second	Quantity of electrons flowing per second
Electrical potential	Volt V	The force that moves electrons within a conductive material	Potential difference across an X-ray tube, acceleration of electrons and quality of X-ray beam
Frequency	Hertz Hz	Number of cycles per second	Electromagnetic radiation

Table 1.5 Radiological units.

Unit	Description	Symbol
kV_p	Maximum energy of X-ray photons	kV_p
mA (mAs)	Electron production in the X-ray tube	mA
keV	Kinetic energy of electrons in X-ray tube	keV
Heat unit	Heat produced at anode ($kV_p \times$ mAs)	HU
Gray	Dose absorbed by a medium	Gy
Sievert	Dose equivalent	Sv
Coulomb/kilogram	Measure of atmospheric exposure	C/kg
Becquerel	Radioactive disintegrations per second	Bq

used in diagnostic imaging. The units are mainly used in assessing and maintaining radiation safety or when discussing the use of the X-ray tube.

kV_p

The potential difference between the cathode and anode in an X-ray tube is measured in kilovolts. This value determines the maximum energy of the X-ray photons emitted that will give the quality and intensity of the beam. In many machines, this value may fluctuate and so the peak value is given (kV_p).

mA/mAs

In the production of X-rays, fast-moving electrons must strike the anode within the X-ray tube. To produce these electrons, an electrical current must be applied to the cathode. This is measured in milliamperes (mA). These electrons could be produced continuously, but this would cause damage to the tube and so the production of electrons is limited to a period of time (exposure time). The exposure time is expressed in mAs or milliamperes per second.

keV

As an electron is accelerated across the tube from the cathode to the anode, it gains kinetic energy. This is measured in keV. The keV will be the same as the kV_p.

Heat units

The production of X-rays produces heat at the anode. The amount of heat is specific to each exposure and can be calculated by multiplying kV_p and mAs together. This is correct only if the voltage and current remain constant throughout the exposure.

Absorbed dose

The dose absorbed by the patient is measured in gray (Gy). This is specific to the patient dose received and will vary according to the exposure used and the region being examined. The absorbed dose is the measurement of the energy absorbed by a medium.

> **1 gray = 1 joule per kilogram**

Dose equivalent

The dose received by designated people working with radiation (dose equivalent) is measured in sieverts (Sv). This measurement is calculated by multiplying the grays received by a quality factor. The quality factor will take into account the different levels of damage caused by radiation and will alter depending on the type of ionising radiations and the energy of the ionising radiation. The dose equivalent is calculated from monitoring devices worn by personnel working with radiation.

Exposure in air

The amount of radiation in the atmosphere can be measured in coulomb/kilogram (C/kg). This measure of radiation can only be used for air and for X-rays or gamma rays within this air. The measure gives the total electric charge formed by ionisation in air. This can be used for X-rays emerging from the tube or the intensity of gamma rays during a scintigraphic examination.

Activity

The final radiographic unit is the becquerel (Bq). Radioactive substances have unstable nuclei and try to change the structure of the nucleus to a more stable form. Each change in structure is called disintegration. The becquerel measures the number of changes per second.

Useful mathematics

Day-to-day radiography involves mathematics. This may be simple addition or multiplication, but can also involve fractions and ratios. As a simple 'aide memoir', this section demonstrates the basic mathematics essential to radiography in Table 1.6, where a and b denote any number and x is any number that you wish to calculate.

Proportions and the inverse square law

Proportions

Measurements can be either directly or indirectly proportional. If two measurements are directly proportional, the ratio of one to the other is constant:

$$\frac{a}{b} = \text{constant}$$

If something is described as being inversely proportional, the factors will be inverted. As one factor increases, the other will decrease, or vice versa:

$$a \times b = \text{constant}$$

Table 1.6 Useful mathematics.

Description	How to do it
Percentage change	$100 \times (b - a/a)$
Percentage of b compared to a	$100b/a$
$x\%$ of a	$(x/100) \times a$
Parts of a fraction	$\dfrac{\text{Numerator}}{\text{Denominator}}\quad \dfrac{a}{b}$
Adding and subtracting fractions	Find a common denominator and then add or subtract the numerators
Multiplying fractions	Multiply numerators and denominators
Dividing fractions	Turn the second fraction upside down and then multiply
Ratio	Demonstrates the relationship between two related measures
	kV : X-rays produced
Decimal	A fraction that has a denominator that can be divided by ten can be shown as a decimal: $5/10 = 0.5$
To calculate x when a and b are known: divide both known numbers by the multiple of x	$ax = b$ $ax/a = b/a$ $x = b/a$
When a known number is added to x: subtract the known number from both sides	$x + a = b$ $x + a - a = b - a$ $x = b - a$
When x is part of a fraction: cross multiply	$x/a = b/c$ $xc = ab$ $x = ab/c$
Cross multiplication	

Inverse square law

The intensity of radiation from a given point is inversely proportional to the square of the distance between that point and the source. This means that the greater the distance between the two points, the weaker the intensity. This plays an important role in radiation safety. The greater the distance between you and the source of radiation, the lower the dose you will receive:

$$I \propto 1/d^2$$

The effect distance has on the exposure is determined by the inverse square law. As the distance of the object from the source increases, the intensity of the radiation will decrease. If you double the distance, the exposure intensity decreases by 4. This can be seen in a similar way using a torch beam. The closer the wall is to the torch beam, the stronger the intensity of the beam against the wall. As you move away from the wall, the beam will be weaker when it hits the wall (Figure 1.1).

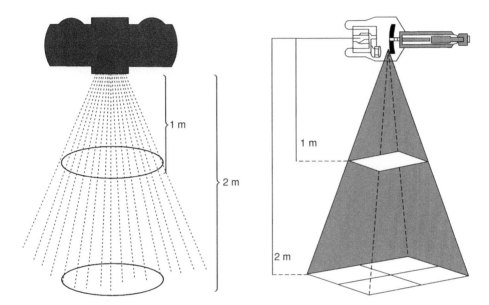

Figure 1.1 The inverse square law.

Revision questions

1 How are mass and matter related?

2 What is weight?

3 List and give examples of three types of energy.

4 What is 30,000 volts in kilovolts?

5 What is 4.5 mA in decimal notation?

6 What name is given to the unit of measure for time?

7 Give the measure of absorbed dose and describe what the measurement demonstrates.

8 Describe the calculation of a becquerel.

9 What is the symbol for a sievert?

(continued)

10 What is a ratio?

11 Add 4/5 to 3/7.

12 Divide 3/10 by 1/8.

13 Work out the following equations:

$$x + 10 = 37$$
$$4x = 24$$
$$x/8 = 3/4$$

14 If a is inversely proportional to b, what will happen to a if b doubles?

15 Using the inverse square law and thinking about an X-ray beam, if you double your object–source distance, what will happen to the intensity and size of the beam when it reaches the object?

Chapter 2

The Principles of Physics Used in Radiography

Chapter contents

Electrostatics – the electric charge
Conductors and insulators
Electricity
Measuring electricity
Types of current
Laws of an electric current
Resistance
Making a circuit – the options
Magnetism
The function and composition of a magnet
Magnetic laws
Electromagnetism – electricity and magnetism in union
Laws of electromagnetic induction
Further reading

Key points

- *Electric charge*: Current × time
- An object becomes charged by the addition or removal of electrons. This can be caused by friction, contact or induction
- *Laws of electricity*: Unlike charges attract, and like charges repel. When an object becomes charged, the charges are spread evenly throughout the object
- Potential energy of electricity is measured in volts (V)
- *Conductors* allow easy flow of electrons
- *Insulators* resist the flow of electrons
- *Currents and circuits*: Electrons flow on the outer surface of a wire. If the wire is in contact at both ends, an electrical circuit is made. The number of electrons flowing in this circuit is measured in amperes (A)
- *Direct current*: Electrons flow in one direction along the conductor

Practical Veterinary Diagnostic Imaging, Second Edition. Suzanne Easton.
© 2012 John Wiley & Sons, Ltd. Published 2012 by Blackwell Publishing Ltd.

- *Alternating current*: Electrons flow in one direction and then in the other direction
- *Magnetism*: A charged moving particle creates a magnetic field. The electrons around the nucleus can be orientated in the same direction using a magnet. Magnetic force will always flow from south to north
- *Magnetic laws*: Opposites attract. Non-magnetic materials can be made magnetic through induction (bringing them into the magnetic field around a magnetic material). Every magnet, however small, will have two poles
- *Electromagnetic induction*: The production of electricity in a magnetic field

Introduction

Although the essential use of electricity is immediately obvious in radiography – the conversion of electrical energy into electromagnetic energy – it also has a subtle role, which is not always considered immediately. Electricity and magnetism are both utilised in the stages leading up to the current and potential difference being available for use in the correct form within the X-ray tube. If the two concepts are not understood and related back to the processes involved in the production of X-rays, understanding of technical and practical procedures will not be possible.

Electrostatics – the electric charge

This imposing term is used to describe the study of electrical charges. These charges are all around and experienced daily. These static electrical charges are seen in many forms – as discharges during storms, and from lightening through to uncontrollable hair after it has been washed! Electric charges are either positive or negative, depending on the material and how they are formed, and like charges always repel each other (Figure 2.1).

Creating an electric charge

An electric charge is created when a negatively charged electron is removed from a positive proton in the nucleus of an atom. The electron removed is a free electron that is very loosely bound to the atom and easy to remove. The simplest way to remove these free electrons is through friction. Other methods of electron removal include heat, which is the method used in the X-ray tube, and induction, the use

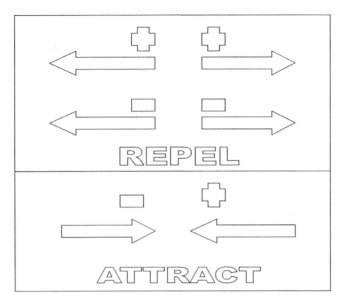

Figure 2.1 Electric charge.

of the electrical field of a charged object to transfer charge to an uncharged object. Charges are of two types: positive and negative. The electron is always negatively charged and the proton is always positively charged. The electron and proton are the smallest units of charge. They have equal magnitude, but opposite signs.

The force between two charges can be calculated using the inverse square law. As the distance between the two charges increases, the force will decrease. However, this will depend on the medium the atom is suspended in and is not constant. Force will be present even when a vacuum separates the atoms.

> **Charge is measured in coulombs (Q).**

One coulomb is equivalent to 6×10^{18} electrons. This is also known as the electromotive force (see Table 2.1).

Table 2.1 Terms related to an electric charge.

Free electrons	Loosely bound electrons in an atom
Positive charge	Created by a proton being separated from an electron
Negative charge	Created by removing an electron from a proton
Force	Between charges, forces will always be equal and opposite. Calculated using the inverse square law
Coulomb	Measure of charge: 1 coulomb $= 6 \times 10^{18}$ electrons

Conductors and insulators

Materials are either conductors or insulators. If the material has free electrons, then it is a conductor. This is usually a material composed of metallic elements. A conductor can be charged through heating, friction or induction. If a conductor is placed in an electrical circuit, then charge will flow through the circuit including the conductor. Examples of conductors include metals such as copper, titanium and aluminium, the earth and the human body.

If a material has very few free electrons, then it will be an insulator. In an insulator, any charge produced on the surface will not move along the material. The charge will remain where it is formed. If the material is placed into a circuit, then no charge will be present, as the material will not allow electrons to flow. Examples of insulators include plastics, rubber, glass and silicon (see Table 2.2).

Table 2.2 Insulators and conductors.

	Electron status	Examples
Insulator	Very few free electrons	Carbon
Conductor	Free electrons present, allowing easy release and movement of electrons	Copper Aluminium

Electricity

A potential difference must occur to achieve current flow. If a piece of wire is joined between a positive and negative point, a potential difference is formed. If a potential difference is present across a piece of wire, then weakly bound electrons will flow through the wire. This is an electrical current.

Measuring electricity

Electricity is measured in volts. This is the potential difference within the circuit, which must be present if a current is to flow.

Volts = joules/coulomb

Two points within a circuit have a potential difference of 1 volt if 1 joule of work is done for every coulomb of electricity passing between the two points.

Every part of a circuit has a maximum potential difference that it is able to produce. This is called the electromotive force. This is measured in volts in the same way as potential difference.

The power of electricity is measured in watts (W). One watt is equal to 1 ampere of current flowing through an electric potential of 1 volt. Household appliances usually need about 500–1000 W to work effectively. An X-ray machine usually needs 30–100 kW of power to work efficiently.

> **Watts = amperes × voltage**

Types of current

Current takes two forms: either alternating or direct. In a circuit with a direct current, the electrons flow in one direction only. This provides a continuous flow that is demonstrated with a straight waveform on a graph (Figure 2.2). The distance between the time axis and the horizontal line of the current will determine the magnitude of the current.

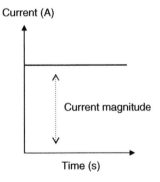

Current (A)

Current magnitude

Time (s)

Figure 2.2   Waveform generated by a direct current.

Alternating current will produce a sinusoidal waveform, with the flow of the current fluctuating between two directions (Figure 2.3). The electrons first move in one direction to their maximum 'positive' potential and then in the reverse direction back to the opposite maximum 'negative' potential.

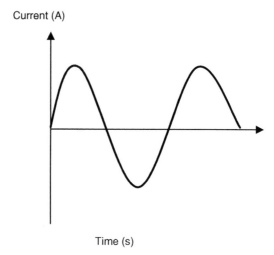

Figure 2.3   Waveform generated by an alternating current.

Laws of an electric current

- An electrical potential difference must be present.
- There must be a complete circuit around which the electrons can flow.
- Current will always flow from positive to negative (whilst electron flow is always from negative to positive).

Resistance

As is already known, a potential difference is necessary to allow current to pass through a conductor. If this potential difference increases, the current increases. If all the physical properties of the conductor remain constant, the potential difference and the current through the material will remain proportional. This is known as Ohm's law.

The units of resistance are measured in ohms (Ω).

If a graph demonstrating resistance is drawn, the gradient will be constant (Figure 2.4). If the physical properties of the conductor are altered, for example temperature changes in a light bulb, the gradient of the graph will alter (Figure 2.5). The resistance through a wire can also be altered if the thickness of the wire is altered. Therefore, the thinner the wire, the greater the resistance.

Potential difference (V)

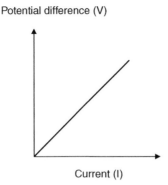

Current (I)

Figure 2.4   Graph to demonstrate resistance.

Potential difference (V)

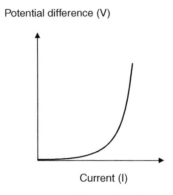

Current (I)

Figure 2.5   Graph to demonstrate resistance when temperature changes occur to the same material.

Making a circuit – the options

When a circuit is designed, a number of different components can be added to alter the function of the circuit or the flow of charge through the circuit. The combinations are extensive; the key elements used in radiography are outlined in Table 2.3.

Magnetism

Magnetic materials exist naturally. The name originates from the discovery of magnetic iron oxide in the village of Magnesia in western Turkey. More recently, alloys have been manufactured that can be made into very strong magnets.

> **Magnetism – the ability of certain materials to attract iron**

Table 2.3 Components of electrical circuits.

Circuit component	Function	Symbol
Battery	Provides a source of electrical potential	
Ammeter	Measures electrical current	
Voltmeter	Measures electrical potential	
Switch	Turns a circuit on or off by providing a means for the electrons to flow in a complete circuit	
Resistor	Slows or reduces the flow of electrons	
Rheostat	A resistor that can have the amount of flow it will allow altered	
Diode	This will restrict the flow of electrons to one direction only	
Transformer	If the current is alternating, the voltage will be increased or decreased by a certain amount	
Capacitor	This is able to store electrical charge. Used in some portable X-ray machines	

The function and composition of a magnet

Every magnet has a pole. This is where the lines of force are most concentrated. An area – the magnetic field – surrounds the poles (Figure 2.6). Poles are always found in pairs.

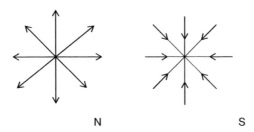

N   S

Figure 2.6   Magnetic lines of force due to north and south poles.

In a magnetic field, force can be exerted on another pole. The simplest example of these forces is seen in a bar magnet (Figure 2.7).

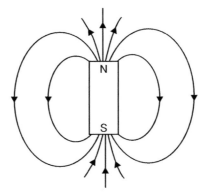

Figure 2.7   Magnetic fields around a bar magnet.

Any charged particle that is moving will have a magnetic field. If the movement of the electron is contained in the nucleus of an atom, the lines of the magnetic field will be perpendicular to the movement of the electron. Electrons will circle the nucleus in either a clockwise or anticlockwise direction. This is known as electron spin. If the wire is circular, the fields will flow in a similar way to those in a bar magnet.

Types of magnets

Magnets fall into two categories: temporary and permanent. A permanent magnet retains its magnetism. The north pole is always the same and will attract other permanent magnets and other magnetic materials.

A temporary magnet loses its magnetism by movement or heating. In some temporary magnets, the force needed to lose magnetism is very small.

Ferromagnetism

Ferromagnetism is the most commonly encountered magnetism in radiography. It is found in transformers and electromagnetic relays, and also in magnetic resonance imaging (MRI) equipment. Ferromagnets are found in large quantities in substances such as iron, nickel and cobalt. In these materials, the atoms are arranged into 'magnetic domains'. Within each domain, the atoms are all pointing in the same direction, although all the domains may not be in a similar direction.

Electromagnetism

An electromagnet is composed of several coils of copper wire around a soft iron core. This coil is called a solenoid. A current is then applied to the wire and an electromagnet is formed.

Magnetic laws

Magnets have a number of laws that are similar to electrostatics and gravity, but are specific to magnets alone.

Attraction and repulsion

The lines of the magnetic field will always exit the magnet from the north pole and flow to the south pole. When placed within the magnetic field of another magnet, like poles will repel and opposing poles will attract.

Existence of poles in pairs

As is the case of the Earth, there will always be two poles. If a magnet is cut or broken in half, two new, smaller magnets will be made, still with two poles (Figure 2.8).

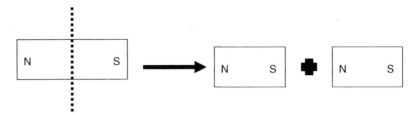

Figure 2.8   The effect of cutting a bar magnet in half.

Magnetic induction

A material that can be easily magnetised, ferromagnetic material, is made up of lots of individual small magnets called dipoles. The dipoles are scattered randomly through the material. If a ferromagnetic material is placed in a magnetic field, the dipoles will arrange themselves in line with the flow of the magnetic field (Figure 2.9).

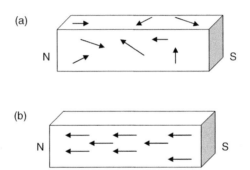

Figure 2.9   Effect of a magnet on the dipoles of ferromagnetic material. (a) Ferromagnetic material with randomly orientated magnetic dipoles. (b) Ferromagnetic material under the influence of a magnet.

Magnetic flux

Magnetic flux is the number of lines of magnetic force passing through a given area. This will vary depending on the density of the material it is passing through. Magnetic flux is described in tesla (T). It is important in the classification of MRI scanners.

> **Magnetic flux is measured in tesla (T).**

Electromagnetism – electricity and magnetism in union

Electromagnetism is the production of electricity by a changing magnetic field. The most basic example of this is the production of electricity using a dynamo. The placing of a conductor into a magnetic field will produce an electromotive force in that conductor. The strength of the magnetic field and the speed of the introduction and removal of the conductor from the magnetic field will alter the size of electromotive force generated (Figure 2.10).

Laws of electromagnetic induction

There are two laws directly related to electromagnetic induction. These can be calculated using Faraday's left hand rule.

Faraday's law

Whenever there is a change in the magnetic flux linked with a circuit, an electromotive force is induced, the strength of which is proportional to the rate of change of the flux through the circuit.

Lenz's law

The direction of the induced current is always such as to oppose the change producing it.

Fleming's left hand rule

Magnetic fields around currents will have an individual anticlockwise magnetic field around every electron. The direction of the magnetic field in relation to the electron flow can be demonstrated using Fleming's left hand rule (Figure 2.10).

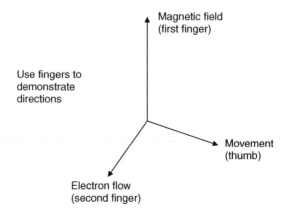

Figure 2.10   Fleming's left hand rule.

Application of the laws in radiography

All of these laws are used within the circuits used to supply the X-ray machine with power. They are used in the transformers and the process of current rectification.

Further reading

Ball, J., Moore, A.D. (1997) *Essential Physics for Radiographers*, 3rd edn. London: Blackwell Publishing Ltd.
A clear introduction to physics for radiographers.

Revision questions

1 How can an electric charge be produced? Give two ways.

2 What is the simplest way to release free electrons?

3 What unit is charge described in?

4 What type of material is used for a conductor?

5 Name two everyday insulators.

6 What must be present to allow a current to flow?

7 What unit is potential difference measured in?

8 Draw a graph to demonstrate the current flow in an alternating current.

9 What is resistance measured in?

10 Does a thin wire have high or low resistance when compared with a thick wire?

11 Draw the symbol for the part of an electric circuit that will allow current to flow only in one direction.

12 If two similar poles of two magnets are brought into close proximity, what will happen?

13 Name the material that could be used for the core of an electromagnet.

14 If a conductor is brought in and out of a magnetic field, what will happen?

15 Name the two laws related to electromagnetic induction.

Chapter 3

Inside the Atom

Chapter contents

Atoms, elements and other definitions
The 'Make-Up' of an atom – atomic structure
Shells and energy
The periodic table
Radioactivity
The effects of an electron changing orbits
Electromagnetic radiation
Frequency and wavelength
Further reading

Key points

- An atom is the smallest unit within an element having all the properties of the element. It is made up of a nucleus containing neutrons and protons surrounded by electrons
- A compound is a combination of different elements
- The periodic table contains details of all elements known to man and provides their proton and nucleon number
- Electrons orbit around the nucleus in shells. These hold a certain number of electrons per shell. If the shell is not complete, the atom will react differently to an atom with a full outer shell
- *Radioactivity* is the emission of particles from an atom with an unstable nucleus with the aim of becoming stable. This emission is called radioactive decay
- *Ionisation* is the interaction of radiation with matter. This involves the removal of an electron from an atom. The ejected electron and the positive atom are called an ion pair
- The electromagnetic spectrum consists of a collection of different types of radiation with a range of energy levels. This includes visible light, radio waves and X-rays
- Constituents of the electromagnetic spectrum move in a wave
- The wavelength is the distance from crest to crest of the wave

Practical Veterinary Diagnostic Imaging, Second Edition. Suzanne Easton.
© 2012 John Wiley & Sons, Ltd. Published 2012 by Blackwell Publishing Ltd.

- The rate of rise and fall of a wave (electromagnetic radiation travels in waves) is called the frequency. It is measured in hertz (Hz)
- If the frequency is high, the wavelength is short

Introduction

The concepts and ideas discussed in this chapter can prove daunting at first. If the concepts are thought of as a miniature solar system, something that can actually be visualised, then the theory will become more manageable and less of a difficulty. The topics in this chapter cannot be shown with photographs or actual props and so a good imagination and acceptance of the work of others is essential.

Atoms will join the theory of matter with ionising radiation to form the base of radiography built in previous chapters to be taken into the following chapters.

Atoms, elements and other definitions

The definitions of an atom, element and other related terms are given in Table 3.1.

Table 3.1   Terms related to atoms.

Term	Symbol	Definition
Atom		The smallest unit of an element that has the specific properties of the element
Atomic or proton number	Z	The number of protons in a nucleus
Nucleon or mass number	A	The total number of protons or neutrons in the nucleus of an atom
Neutron number	N	The number of neutrons within the nucleus
Element	E	A nucleus with a set, known atomic number that cannot be broken down into anything smaller
Compound		The substance formed when two or more elements join together chemically
Isotope		An atom with the same atomic number, but a different atomic mass number and number of neutrons as the given element
Isobar		An atom with the same atomic mass number as the given element, but a different atomic number and number of neutrons in the nucleus
Radioisotope		A nucleus of an atom with particular atomic mass and atomic mass number, which is radioactive

The 'Make-Up' of an atom – atomic structure

The atom is the basic unit involved in the production and use of X-rays. Unless a vacuum has been created, atoms are present in every solid, liquid and gas.

The atomic nucleus

Atoms are composed of a nucleus that contains protons and neutrons. Protons are positively charged. Neutrons have no electrical charge. Neutrons and protons together are termed nucleons. Electrons surround the nucleus of an atom (Figure 3.1).

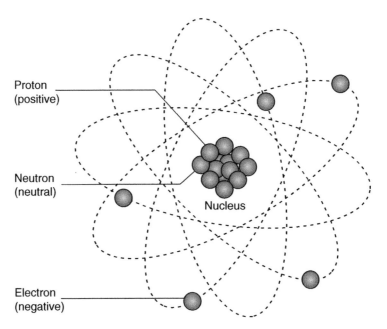

Proton (positive)

Neutron (neutral)

Nucleus

Electron (negative)

Figure 3.1   The structure of an atom.

Protons and neutrons are about 2000 times bigger than electrons. For this reason, the mass of an atom is almost completely made up of the protons and neutrons in its nucleus. The total number of protons and neutrons in the nucleus is known as the mass number. Forces known as short-range forces hold the nucleus together. These are very strong forces. The energy used in keeping the nucleus together is called binding energy.

If the nucleus was scaled to match the centre spot of a football pitch, the electron shells would start at the perimeter of the pitch and the outer orbits would be found several miles beyond this.

Shells and energy

The electrons orbit around the nucleus in different planes; these planes are called shells. The shells are called K, L, M, N, O and P. Normally, the number of electrons orbiting the nucleus equals the number of protons found in the nucleus (Table 3.2). The shells nearest the nucleus will always be the first to be completely filled. This is because they have lower energy levels and are easier to fill. If there are not enough electrons to fill the shell, then the odd electrons will be found in the outermost shell. Each shell has a maximum number of electrons that it can hold, before the next shell is entered. If the outer shell is full, the atom will be stable. If the outer shell is not full, the atom will attempt to gain electrons to fill the outer shell. This will make the atom unstable. Elements such as copper or tungsten, which are good conductors of heat and electricity, will have a single electron in the outer shell, which leaves easily and can act as a free electron.

Table 3.2   Number of electrons in atomic shells.

Shell number	Shell letter	Maximum number of electrons
1	K	2
2	L	8
3	M	18
4	N	32

The maximum number of electrons in each shell is calculated using $2n^2$, where n equals the shell number.

The periodic table

All elements known to man are arranged in the periodic table. This table displays all the elements in groups according to their chemical and physical properties. Group I is composed of the alkali metals (excluding hydrogen), which combine easily with oxygen and react violently with water. Elements in Group VIII are called the noble gases. These do not react with other elements easily. By convention, the periodic table will show the atomic mass and atomic number of every element. The atomic number will always be above the symbol for the element and the mass number will always be below the element symbol (Figure 3.2). Using the periodic table, the number of electrons, protons and neutrons in an atom can be calculated.

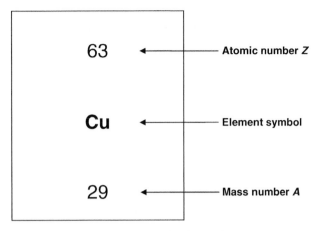

Figure 3.2   Single unit from the periodic table (copper).

Proton or atomic number

Symbol: Z

The atomic number represents the number of protons in the nucleus of an atom. An atom with just one proton is hydrogen. If the nucleus contains eight protons, then the atom is oxygen, and if it has 56 protons, then it is barium. These numbers will be found in the periodic table and can be used in determining how the atom will react to X-ray interactions.

Nucleon or mass number

Symbol: A

This number identifies the number of nucleons in the nucleus, which is the number of protons plus neutrons in the nucleus. By subtracting the proton number from the nucleon number, the number of neutrons in the nucleus will be identified. Barium is used in contrast medium and has a nucleon number of 137 and a proton number of 56. This means that barium has 56 protons and 81 neutrons in its each atom.

Isotopes

The number of neutrons in a nucleus can vary depending on a number of factors. This can occur either naturally or artificially. One such isotope is carbon-14. Carbon has a proton number of 6, but the nucleon number may be 11, 12, 13 or 14. Each has a different number of neutrons. Carbon-14 is used to date historical artefacts as it decays at a known rate, and carbon-12 is used as a baseline to determine the atomic mass of other elements. Some isotopes are stable, while others are radioactive depending on the proton to neutron ratio.

Radioactivity

Any nucleus that is unstable is said to be radioactive. The nucleus will attempt to change the internal structure to a more stable form, sometimes resulting in the ejection of a charged particle from the nucleus. Every time the nucleus changes its structure, it is called a radioactive disintegration or transformation. This may result in a change to the atomic number, the atomic mass number or both. If the atomic number is changed, then the resulting element will be different. It is not possible to predict which atom in a sample will change its internal structure; the disintegration of an atom is random event.

Elements with a high mass number are more likely to consist of isotopes and therefore undergo a change in nucleus structure. This is because these elements have atoms with far more neutrons than protons. This excess in neutrons will lead to instability.

The effects of an electron changing orbits

Although electrons are usually found in the orbits surrounding the nucleus with the innermost shells filled, this is not always the case. Protons are positively charged (+1) and electrons are negatively charged (−1). A balanced atom has the same number of electrons and protons. The charges create a force known as binding energy, which holds the electrons in orbit around the nucleus. This type of atom is stable. If an electron is removed from the atom, the protons will outweigh the negative electrons and the resulting atom will have a positive charge. An electron within an atom can undergo a collision or interaction at any time. This event will alter the energy level of the electron, producing either excitation or ionisation. The unit of electromagnetic radiation (EMR) produced during this interaction is known as a photon or quantum.

Excitation

Interactions can occur that will give the electron enough energy to move from one orbit to an outer orbit. This is known as excitation. This 'excited' electron is then able to return to its original orbit, releasing a photon of EMR as it does so. This process is used in thermoluminescent dosemeters.

Ionisation

Ionisation occurs when an electron is subjected to enough energy to remove it from the atom completely. The more the protons found in the nucleus, the higher the binding energy required to remove the electron. The closer the shell is to the nucleus, the higher the binding energy. When the electron is 'free', it has a kinetic energy (Figure 3.3). The ejected electron and the positive atom are called an ion pair. Atoms can be ionised by X-ray photons. Damage to cells can occur if the ionisation process occurs in DNA. As the X-rays overcome the binding energy of the electrons, changes to the chemical structure of the cells can occur, causing permanent damage.

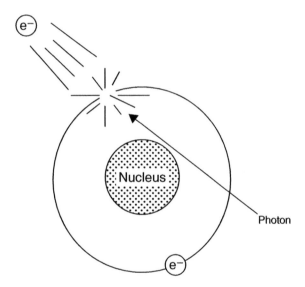

Figure 3.3   The effects of ionisation on the position of an electron in an atom.

Electromagnetic radiation

The EMR spectrum consists of waves of vibrations of electric and magnetic fields, all travelling with the same speed. This is the speed of light in a vacuum, which is 3×10^8 metres per second. As it is always the same, it is used as a constant (C). The waves differ in their frequency and wavelength. They will always travel in straight lines at 90° to each other, which is important for the inverse square law. The EMR includes a range of radiation types including radio waves, infrared light, microwaves and X-rays (Table 3.3 and Figure 3.4). Outside a vacuum, EMR will interact with matter – a property that we use in diagnostic imaging.

Table 3.3   The electromagnetic spectrum.

Wavelength	Type	Production	Example
$>10^{-4}$	Radio	Electrons oscillating in wires	Radio frequency pulses in magnetic resonance imaging
7×10^{-7} to 10^{-4}	Infrared	Hot objects	Heat transfer from the anode in the X-ray tube
4×10^{-7} to 7×10^{-7}	Visible	Very hot objects	Detected with the eye; viewing radiographs
10^{-9} to 4×10^{-7}	Ultraviolet	Arcs and gas discharges	Intensifying screens
10^{-12} to 10^{-8}	X-rays	Electrons hitting metal target	Used in diagnostic imaging
$<10^{-10}$	γ-rays	Radioactive nuclei	Used in nuclear medicine and in the treatment of carcinoma

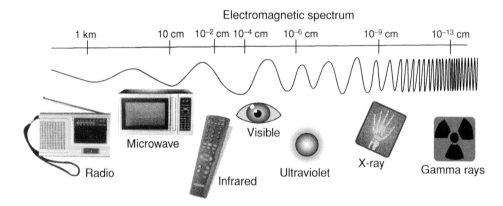

Figure 3.4   Electromagnetic spectrum.

Frequency and wavelength

Wavelength and frequency relate to any form of wave. In the context of radiography, this is the electromagnetic spectrum.

Wavelength (λ)

The wavelength is the distance between two consecutive peaks or troughs during the movement of a wave of any type.

Frequency (v)

Frequency is the number of cycles of the wave passing a fixed point per second and is measured in hertz (Hz). This is inversely proportional to the wavelength.

The smaller the wavelength, the higher the frequency or energy of the wave.

As frequency and wavelength are inversely proportional, an increase in wavelength will result in a decrease in frequency. To remember these changes, think of trying to run taking large strides and how it is not possible. Your stride size relates to the wavelength and your speed of movement to the frequency.

> **A radio wave has a long wavelength and a low frequency.**
> **X-rays have a short wavelength and a high frequency.**
> **X-rays with a shorter wavelength will have more penetrating power than those with a long wavelength.**

Planck's constant

X-ray photons will travel at the speed of light, and will either exist and have a velocity or will not exist at all. The energy of an X-ray photon is directly proportional to the frequency of the photon. This is Planck's constant.

> **E (eV) = h × f**
> **Photon energy (eV) = Planck's constant × Photon frequency**

Further reading

Graham, D.T., Cloke, P. (2003) *Principles of Radiological Physics*, 4th edn. London: Churchill Livingstone.
An in-depth introduction to medical physics with clear presentation and application to practice. This is human based, but the principles are the same.
There are a number of sources of the periodic table, and it is worth finding a copy and looking at all of the elements used in radiography, where they sit within the table and what properties they exhibit. This will help to identify why they are selected for the specific use.

> **Revision questions**
>
> 1 What are the small discrete packets of electromagnetic radiation called?
>
> 2 What does the atomic number of an atom depend upon?
>
> *(continued)*

3 What is the term given to the positively charged particles contained within the nucleus of an atom?

4 What is a molecule?

5 How many electrons should there be in the innermost shell of an atom?

6 If an atom gains or loses one or more electrons, what is it called?

7 Name two parts of the electromagnetic spectrum.

8 What does the nucleus of an atom contain?

9 If the frequency of a wave is high, does it have a long or short wavelength?

10 What is the unit measure of frequency?

Chapter 4

The X-ray Tube

Chapter contents

The tube housing
The cathode
The anode
The line focus principle
The anode-heel effect
The stator assembly
Tube rating
How to look after your X-ray tube
Further reading

Key points

- The cathode is the negative part of the X-ray tube and produces electrons through the heating of the tungsten filament
- Electrons are collected in a focussing cup that controls the electron stream through electrostatic focussing
- The filament size regulates the size of the focal spot. The smaller the focal spot, the smaller the penumbra generated
- The anode is the positive end of the X-ray tube with a tungsten target where fast-moving electrons are rapidly decelerated, resulting in the formation of X-rays
- The target is angled to provide a greater surface area for the electrons to strike and rotates to spread the heat loading over a larger area, preventing overheating
- The cathode and anode are supported in a glass envelope containing a vacuum, allowing maximum efficiency to the acceleration of the electrons
- X-rays are produced as bremsstrahlung and characteristic radiation with 99% of the energy produced in the form of heat
- The glass envelope is surrounded by oil, lead and an aluminium casing

Practical Veterinary Diagnostic Imaging, Second Edition. Suzanne Easton.
© 2012 John Wiley & Sons, Ltd. Published 2012 by Blackwell Publishing Ltd.

- The electrons are accelerated from the cathode to the anode when a potential difference is applied across the tube. This potential difference ranges from 40 to approximately 90 kV in veterinary radiography
- X-rays exit the tube through an opening in the lead that contains aluminium to remove the very-low-energy X-rays. The X-rays are emitted in all directions, but the tube window only limits the use of X-rays to those moving in a forward direction
- Every X-ray tube has a maximum amount of electrical energy it is able to receive, which is known as the tube loading

Introduction

The X-ray tube is continuously evolving and becoming more efficient over time. It uses the electrons produced at the cathode to produce X-rays as they interact with the tungsten at the anode. The key components of the rotating anode X-ray tube are (Figure 4.1):

- Tube housing
- Glass envelope
- Cathode or filament assembly
- Anode
- Stator assembly
- X-ray port and collimator

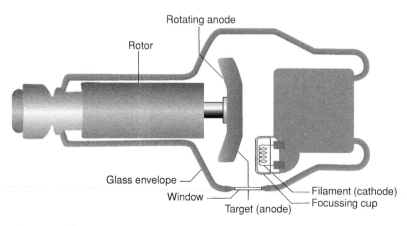

Figure 4.1   Schematic diagram of an X-ray tube.

The tube housing

The cathode and anode are contained, supported and protected by the structures known collectively as the X-ray tube housing. The X-ray tube is supported through the use of fixed or mobile supports. The X-ray tube and its associated supports should never be used to maintain patient position or as fixing points when ties are being used. The cables or supports are not designed for this purpose and their use can result in injury to the patient or operator, damage to the equipment or non-diagnostic images.

The tube housing is made of steel or aluminium with a painted protective coat to allow easy cleaning. The cover has mounting rings to allow attachment to the tube support and sealed sockets for the attachment of the high-tension cables. The position of the sockets will alter depending on the support used for the tube and the layout of the X-ray room.

The housing is marked with the date of manufacture as well as electrical characteristics. It will also indicate the position of the anode focal point.

Glass envelope

The anode and cathode are contained within a Pyrex glass envelope. The glass is usually made of borosilicate, which is strong, does not expand greatly when heated and provides electrical insulation. In high-power X-ray machines, the tube may be made of metal or ceramic, providing greater strength and mechanical stability. The glass envelope is able to withstand the heat produced during the production of X-rays, which is usually above $3000°C$. The envelope also needs to be strong enough to support the anode, cathode and the supporting circuits. It also needs to provide electrical insulation between the cathode and anode. This glass envelope has had all the molecules removed to provide a vacuum. The vacuum prevents unwanted collisions occurring before the electrons reach the anode. The cathode and anode are securely fastened to the glass tube to maintain their position.

Oil

The glass envelope is surrounded by oil. The oil will take heat away from the tube. It will also prevent the tube from overheating and provides electrical insulation. The oil will expand as it heats. A diaphragm within the envelope will move outwards without altering the pressure within the oil. Once the diaphragm reaches its maximum limit, a micro-switch will be tripped and further X-ray production will be prevented until the oil has cooled and the diaphragm has released the micro-switch.

Lead lining

The cover is lined with lead to reduce the leakage of radiation. This covers the whole of the inside of the housing except for a small area called the tube port. The leakage from the X-ray tube housing should be below 1 mGy h^{-1} at 1 m when operating at its maximum setting with the collimators closed. The practice radiation protection advisor will check this during their annual visit.

Tube port

The X-rays produced in an X-ray tube will travel in all directions. Only the X-rays that come directly from the target to form the cone of radiation make up the useful beam, otherwise known as the primary beam. The primary beam will pass through the tube port and exit the X-ray tube. The tube port is made of plastic or beryllium, ground as thinly as possible. This will absorb all the low-energy X-rays from the primary beam that are not useful. Beryllium is used as it has a proton number of 4 and will only absorb the very-low-energy X-rays produced. All the other X-rays produced will have their path altered or stopped by the lead shielding surrounding the X-ray tube (Figure 4.2).

Beam filtration

The X-ray beam is filtered in two ways: inherent and added filtration.

Inherent filtration is the filtration that occurs due to the components of the X-ray tube and is measured in aluminium equivalent in millimetres. Added filtration is the aluminium filters placed over the tube port to remove low-energy X-rays from the primary beam. These low-energy X-rays do not play any useful role in the production of the image. Total filtration is the combination of inherent and added filtration. The total filtration should not be less than 2.5 mm aluminium equivalent and is the measured equivalent of the tube, housing, collimator and any additional filters.

Further filtration can be added by the use of copper filters. Filtration will reduce patient dose during some procedures by the removal of additional lower energy X-ray photons.

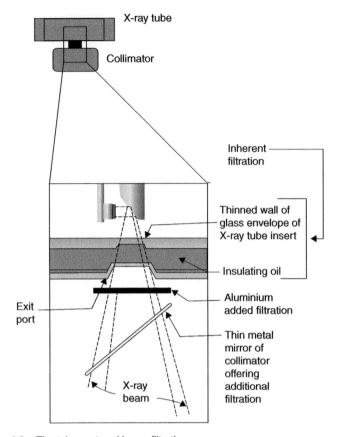

Figure 4.2   The tube port and beam filtration.

The cathode

The cathode is also known as the filament and serves as the negative electrode of the X-ray tube that is necessary to allow the movement of electrons. It is also the source of electrons necessary for the production of X-rays. The cathode is composed of a wire filament made from tungsten. Tungsten has a high atomic number and a very high melting point of 3410°C. Tungsten is used because of the following properties:

- It is dense.
- It is hard.
- It is easy to shape for use.
- It produces electrons easily when heated.
- It has a low vapour pressure.
- It has a high melting point.

The filament of an X-ray tube works in a similar way to the filament in a toaster. In a toaster, the filament is heated until it emits heat; in an X-ray tube, the filament is heated until it emits electrons. This process of electron production is known as thermionic emission. Using the basic principles described earlier, the use of heat is a very effective method of producing free electrons. Increasing or decreasing the current passing through the filament alters its temperature. This is through alteration of the mA.

When the X-ray unit is first switched on, the filament is held at a low temperature; the temperature is not high enough for thermionic emission to occur. When the machine is placed in the 'prepare' position, the filament is heated to the correct level to allow thermionic emission to produce the necessary electrons. This prevents electron production occurring until the unit is ready for exposures to be made. The temperature of the filament is maintained at an exact temperature during exposure so that the correct number of electrons for the mA selected are produced (see Figure 4.3).

Cathode	Responsible for electron production
	Composed of the filament and the focussing cup

The focussing cup

The focussing cup contains the filament. Since all of the electrons are negatively charged, they automatically repel each other. This means that the electrons will spread out as they are accelerated towards the anode and some may miss the anode altogether. The focussing cup is negatively charged and will control the electron stream to ensure all electrons strike the anode. The focussing cup is made of molybdenum or nickel to ensure stability as the heat within the X-ray tube increases (Figure 4.4).

Dual-focus tubes

On some machines in use for veterinary work, the focal spot size can be altered. This can be especially useful when examining the main torso of horses and cattle. Focal spot sizes are usually described as fine and broad. The fine focal spot size will provide better resolution to the resultant image with more sharpness caused by a reduction in the penumbra effect. However, this does mean that the overall coverage is also reduced.

The reduction in penumbra is because of the smaller size of the electron stream emerging from the focussing cup and striking the

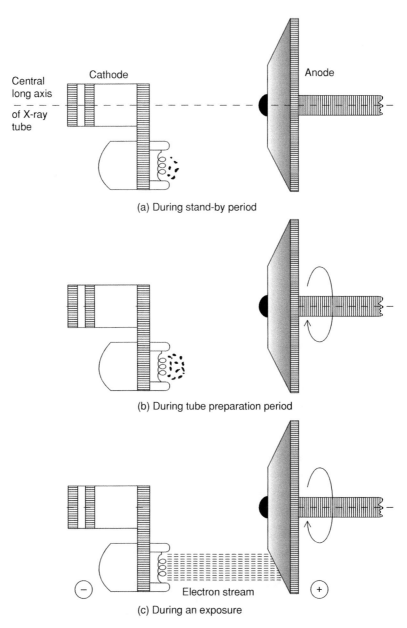

Central
long axis
of X-ray
tube

Cathode

Anode

(a) During stand-by period

(b) During tube preparation period

Electron stream

(c) During an exposure

Figure 4.3   The stages in the preparation of the X-ray tube ready for exposure.

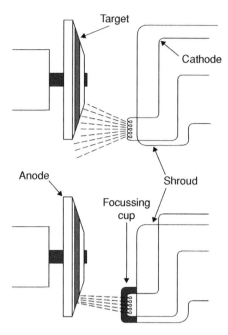

Figure 4.4 Function of the focussing cup.

anode. The broad focus is especially useful in large animal imaging, as the filament will function with an mA above 400 mA. This will spread the heat on the anode as the electrons strike and allow reduction of the exposure times used.

The length of the filament with fine focus is 0.1–0.5 mm and with broad focus is from 0.4 to 1.2 mm. However, the filament size will alter from one machine to another.

Fine focus	Small filament size
	Reduction in penumbra
	Good for small animal radiography
Broad focus	Larger filament size
	Higher mA selection possible
	Good for large animal radiography

The anode

The anode is the positive part of the X-ray tube. It contains a target that is made from solid tungsten. In machines that are capable of producing multiple exposures with a high exposure, the anode will rotate. In these units, the tungsten is mounted on molybdenum or graphite to allow easier rotation of the anode.

There are two types of X-ray tube anodes: stationary anode and rotating anode.

> *Anode*:
> **Positive part of the X-ray tube**
> **Contains the target that will be struck by electrons to facilitate the production of X-rays**
> **Supports the target**
> **Removes heat from the target area**

Stationary anode

Stationary anodes are found in portable and some mobile machines where a high tube current and power are not necessary. The anode is fixed in a block of copper to dissipate the heat away from the target. To reduce the heat as much as possible, the anode is placed at an angle to the electrons striking the surface. This means that there is a larger area for the electrons to strike whilst still keeping the focal spot size to a minimum. The angle of the target in a machine with a stationary anode is about 16°. The X-rays are produced in a small area measuring approximately 4 mm^2, which causes rapid temperature rises, limiting the load on the tube (Figure 4.5).

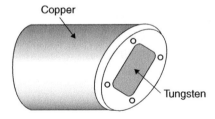

Figure 4.5   Stationary anode.

Rotating anode

This is used in machines that can produce a high output. The anode disc is 7-mm thick and between 55 and 100 mm in diameter with a tungsten–rhenium target area. Rhenium is added in a small amount (5–10%) to reduce damage to the surface of the anode. The anode rotates at approximately 50 rotations each second (3000–10,000 rpm) and the electrons strike the centre of the target strip. The target area measures about 9 cm with an area of 1200 mm^2. This allows the heat to spread during the production of X-rays. This gives a very small focal spot whilst giving a greater area for the heat to be dispersed. This will prevent the pitting and crazing damage that the heat will eventually cause (Figure 4.6).

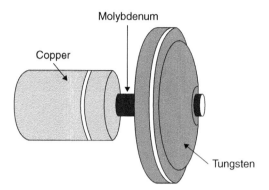

Figure 4.6   Rotating anode.

Some high-capacity machines may have the tungsten target embedded into a molybdenum disc with a graphite backing to dissipate heat further and to reduce the weight of the target.

> **Focal spot:**
> **The area on the target being struck by electrons.**
> **If the target angle is reduced, the focal spot will be reduced.**
>
> **Effective focal spot:**
> **This is the size of the focal spot used in the production of a radiographic image.**

The line focus principle

Penumbra

Penumbra occurs due to the divergence of the primary beam. If a small focal spot (fine focus) is used, then the X-ray beam will be formed in a very small area. This gives the latent image in great detail, but increases the amount of heat received by one small area of the anode. Penumbra will give a slightly irregular or unsharp image. This is more apparent in an image that has been produced using a double-sided emulsion and two intensifying screens. Penumbra may also occur with alteration of the collimation or alteration in the object–film distance.

By ensuring that the object is always as close to the film as possible, penumbra from distance can be reduced to a minimum (Figure 4.7).

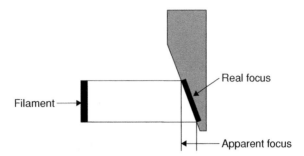

Figure 4.7   The line focus principle.

Focal spot size

The focal spot is the area on the anode where the electrons strike. The focal spot is angled to decrease the area so that it is possible for the electrons to strike. The smallest possible focal spot is achieved with a 7° angle, although the average is nearer to 20°. With a smaller focal spot, less divergence of the primary beam occurs, giving an image of a higher quality, as there is less distortion. The distortion would appear as very fine blurring or a reduction in the image quality. It would also reduce the amount of heat produced at the anode. The size of the focal spot is discussed in the international standard BS EN 60336:2005, and manufacturers must abide by this standard when manufacturing X-ray tubes.

The anode-heel effect

The anode-heel effect occurs because of the absorption of X-rays by the heel of the anode. It means that images on the anode side of the radiograph will have a reduction in sharpness due to the reduction in the intensity of the X-ray beam. The heel effect increases with a reduction in anode angle and can cause a reduction in intensity of the beam by up to 45%. Usually, the steeper the angle of the anode, the more noticeable the effect (Figure 4.8).

The stator assembly

The stator assembly controls the rotation of the anode. This is linked to the exposure switch, ensuring that the anode only rotates when required and is stopped as soon as the exposure has been made. This

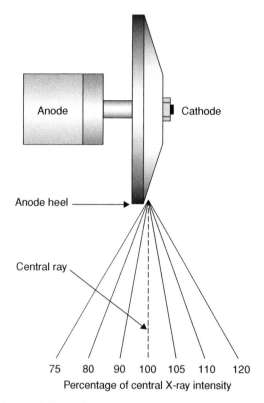

Anode

Cathode

Anode heel

Central ray

75   80   90   100   105   110   120
Percentage of central X-ray intensity

Figure 4.8   The anode-heel effect.

preserves the life of the bearing made of lead and silver, which has a life of approximately 1000 hours. The stem connecting the anode to the stator assembly is made of molybdenum to reduce the transmission of heat along the stem.

Tube rating

The tube rating is the maximum amount of electrical energy (the load) that may be applied to the tube by a single exposure, a series of exposures or a single long exposure without causing damage or over-heating to any part of the tube assembly. The maximum temperature determines the tube rating each part of its structure can reach before damage will occur. The damage that can be caused includes pitting or cracking of the anode surface, damage to the cathode if the anode becomes too hot and starts to release electrons, melting of the target or the deposition of tungsten within the glass envelope.

Rating is measured in the heat unit (HU), which is calculated by multiplying the kV_p with the mAs, and a correction factor depending on the generator type. The manufacturer will supply this. The manufacturer will also give details of the maximum load that can be applied by a single exposure using different kV_p values. This is in the form of a chart showing maximum exposure factors at certain kV_p levels. These charts should be used in conjunction with the anode cooling charts that provide the cooling time needed by the anode after an exposure.

How to look after your X-ray tube

Extension of the tube filament life

- *Careful selection of mA*: Consistent use of a very high mA will eventually damage the filament.
- *Minimising 'prepare' time*: When the X-ray tube is in the 'prepare stage', the filament is supplied with a higher current that will evaporate the tungsten.
- Minimise careless and rough handling of the tube to protect the filament.

Prevention of damage to the anode

- Always remember to warm up your tube with gradually increasing exposure factors before an examination requiring very high exposures is performed. If this is not carried out, the high temperature associated with a large exposure may crack the anode.
- Ensure that fine or broad focus is correctly selected to prevent overheating of the anode.

General care

- Check for oil leakage on a regular basis to prevent heat damage to the tube.
- Full understanding of the limitations of the machine will extend its life.
- Keeping high exposures to a minimum will reduce the tungsten deposits within the tube.
- Choose the tube most suitable for the work you intend to use it for.

Further reading

Bushong, S. (2004) *Radiological Science for Technologists: Physics, Biology and Protection*, 8th edn. St Louis: Elsevier-Mosby.
An excellent all-round physics textbook with very good diagrams to help with the understanding of the structure of the X-ray tube.

Revision questions

1 Describe the structure of the cathode.

2 How are broad and fine foci determined?

3 What function does the focussing cup have?

4 How are the electrons necessary for the production of X-rays produced?

5 What is the difference between a stationary and rotating anode?

6 What is the focal spot?

7 What is the effective focal spot?

8 Give three parts of the tube housing.

9 Describe three ways that the X-ray tube can be protected.

10 What is the tube rating?

Chapter 5

Diagnostic Equipment

Chapter contents

The X-ray circuit
What is seen from the outside?
High-voltage generators
Rectification
Mains supply switch
Primary circuit
Operating console
Filament circuit – control of the mA
High-tension circuit – provision of kV
Making an exposure – switches, timers and interlocks
Types of X-ray machines
Health and safety requirements
Power rating
Further reading

Key points

- The X-ray circuit is made up of the generator, filament circuit, high-tension circuit and the primary circuit
- A generator provides a constant voltage supply to the X-ray machine
- Rectification provides a current that does not alternate
- Half-wave rectification eliminates the negative part of a waveform
- Full-wave rectification provides a constant positive voltage across the X-ray tube
- Three-phase power provides current that never drops to zero
- High-frequency generators provide a near-constant waveform with a high frequency
- An X-ray machine can be isolated using the mains supply switch
- The primary circuit contains the meters necessary to determine the exposure factors being set prior to the exposure being made
- Mains voltage compensation is essential to maintain the voltage at a constant level during an examination

Practical Veterinary Diagnostic Imaging, Second Edition. Suzanne Easton.
© 2012 John Wiley & Sons, Ltd. Published 2012 by Blackwell Publishing Ltd.

- The operating console demonstrates the mains voltage compensation, kV selected, mA and time selected and provides a local on/off switch
- A transformer increases or decreases an alternating current
- The filament circuit controls the mA. This provides the current necessary to heat the cathode
- The high-tension circuit controls the kV supply to the X-ray tube
- Timers terminate the exposure after a pre-selected period of time
- Interlocks prevent an exposure being made if the results damage the X-ray tube or movement of a piece of equipment causes injury to the operator
- The power rating of an X-ray machine is described in kilowatts

Introduction

The equipment for the production of X-rays entails more than just the X-ray tube. A circuit is necessary to supply the electricity to allow the function of the X-ray tube. This chapter concentrates on the parts that make up the rest of the X-ray 'machine' (Figure 5.1).

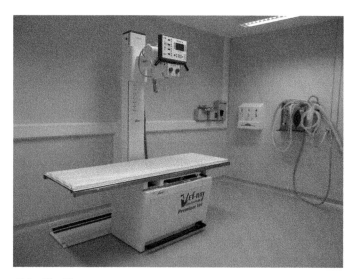

Figure 5.1   The X-ray room.

The X-ray circuit

The X-ray circuit is made up of a number of constituent parts. In isolation they perform no useful function, but when joined together, the end result is the production of X-rays. The constituent parts may be compacted in a portable machine for easy use and mobility, or may be found in separate rooms if the machine is fixed. The X-ray circuit should not be subjected to 'DIY' maintenance. The parts are delicate and easily damaged and, most importantly, use very high voltages that may prove fatal if a qualified engineer does not carry out maintenance.

What is seen from the outside?

The circuit is usually contained within a non-descript box-shaped unit. If the machine is fixed, the generator will be visible as a large box off to one side of the room or under the table. These types of machines will also have a fixed console, from which the exposure factors can be set and the exposure actually made. These consoles will also have the mains voltage compensator and other meters essential to the function of the X-ray machine. Portable and mobile machines will have the generator and the console contained either on the tube mounting or on the main body of the machine separated from the tube by an extendable supporting arm. The X-ray tube itself is fairly small in comparison to the rest of the 'machine'. In mobile and fixed machines, the tube is usually round in shape, supported on a movable arm. In portable machines, the X-ray tube may be incorporated into the body of the 'machine' with no visible, specific tube region.

High-voltage generators

The generator is responsible for converting the mains voltage supply into a form that is suitable for use in the X-ray machine. In the X-ray tube, electrons cannot be accelerated from the anode to the cathode without causing major damage to the tube. For this reason, the current entering the tube must flow in one direction only.

The electrical energy used in a generator is derived from mechanical energy. This effect will produce a kilovoltage with a suitable waveform. The current supplied by the mains is alternating. This means that the average voltage is zero. To overcome this and provide a constant voltage from a constantly reversing current, rectification is necessary.

Generator	Provides a constant voltage supply to the X-ray machine

Rectification

Rectification will provide a current that does not alternate. The curve of a sine wave is known to fluctuate evenly between positive and negative during one cycle. If a rectifier is placed into the circuit, during the positive portion of the AC waveform, the rectifier will allow electrons to flow and pass through the X-ray tube. During the negative part of the waveform, the rectifier will not conduct and no current will flow. Rectification occurs through the use of a diode, a small electrical component that allows flow of current in one direction only.

Mains supply switch

This switch will isolate all equipment in an emergency and when the unit is shut down (Figure 5.2). It contains a fuse (short piece of wire) that will melt if an abnormally high current flows through the fuse. The switch handle is connected to a copper rod with connectors. The connectors must make contact with the circuitry of the generator to allow the current to flow. The switch also has a spring to prevent accidental use.

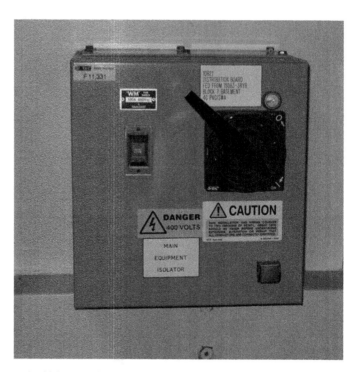

Figure 5.2   Mains supply switch.

Primary circuit

The primary circuit contains all of the meters necessary to determine the exposure being set prior to an exposure being made. These meters must not affect the reading while they measure the flow of electrons. The internal resistance of the circuit is kept to a minimum to ensure accurate readings.

Voltmeter

This meter measures the potential difference in kV that will be applied to the tube during an exposure. An auto-transformer made up of coils with a terminal stud will control the kV. When the switch on the control panel is turned on, contact is made with a stud, which determines the kV selected.

kV compensator

The kV compensator will maintain the kV selected, irrespective of the mA selected. The mA must be selected before the kV.

Mains voltage compensation

During the normal working day, the mains voltage supply will fluctuate. A lift being used in the building or a lunchtime rush to use all the kettles in the vicinity can cause such a fluctuation. The length and width of cables used will also affect the voltage supplied to the unit due to resistance. This must be overcome, otherwise the kV selected will be incorrect and the resultant image will be incorrectly exposed. To maintain a constant voltage supply to the X-ray machine, the incoming mains supply is passed over a bank of resistors to give a constant voltage. In some machines, this can be altered through the alignment of a needle with a fixed point on a meter. This compensation may be automatic in some larger fixed units.

Operating console

The control panel will have a reading to show the kV selected, another to show the mA or time or mAs selected (Figure 5.3). The mains voltage compensator selector and reading/indicator will also be found on the control panel. An indication of when an exposure is being made will also be found on the control panel either in the form of a light or a buzzer. Awareness and familiarity of the operating console for your particular machine is essential if errors in exposure selection are to be avoided.

Modern machines have pre-set, anatomically programmed exposure values, which are stored on a microprocessor. This stores a

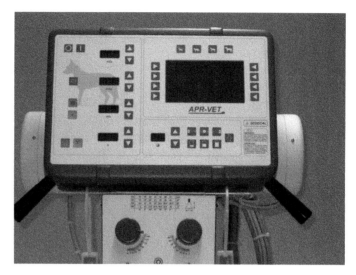

Figure 5.3   Control panel.

list of suitable exposure factors for the practice; however, care and consideration should be taken when using the exposure settings to ensure the exposure selected is suitable for the patient.

Dose area product (DAP) meter

Modern machines have an integrated meter to record the dose received by each patient during each examination. This allows the practitioner to measure the dose and ensure it is within the recommended dose reference level. Whilst this is not required for veterinary patients, it is a good practice to adopt to ensure the dose is kept to a minimum and collimation is accurate. The DAP meter displays the dose given to each patient in milligrays (mGy); this should be recorded and the meter reset after each use.

Filament circuit – control of the mA

The filament circuit will provide the current to the filament in the X-ray tube. It provides the small current (mA) necessary to heat the cathode. Changing the number of resistors that the current flows through alters the filament current. There will be one resistor for each mA value that is available. As the mA increases, the temperature of the filament increases and so the number of electrons available increases.

Space charge compensator

A space charge compensator will maintain the mA, irrespective of the kV selected. If this were not present, the alteration of kV would reduce the mA and the number of electrons produced. Radiography needs to be performed using the highest mA possible, irrespective of the kV selected, and so the space charge compensator is essential.

High-tension circuit – provision of kV

The high-tension circuit provides the kV necessary for an exposure. This usually involves a 1:1000 or 1:1500 step-up transformer. The kV supplied to the X-ray tube can be adjusted by altering the transformer tappings used. A rectifier will ensure that the current will only flow in one direction – from the cathode to the anode. The higher the kV selected, the higher the energy level of the X-rays produced.

Making an exposure – switches, timers and interlocks

The making of an exposure is controlled by the formation and maintenance of a circuit through the X-ray machine. This control can be through switches, timers or interlocks. Whenever an exposure is made, there is a visible or audible (or preferably both) indication that the exposure has been made. This may include movement of the mA indicator, noise from a buzzer or other audible noise.

Primary switching

During an exposure, the power will surge. To prevent damage and reverse flow (arcing) through the X-ray tube when the current is applied, switching must be present and accurate. The accuracy of the switches is improved through the use of electromagnets.

Timers

Timers must be accurate, as they will allow the exposure to be made for the required length of time. Exposure will be terminated when the circuit to the tube is opened manually by releasing the exposure button or when the timer terminates the exposure. The most basic timer uses a clockwork mechanism utilising a tensed spring that unwinds during the time selected. Electronic timers are more accurate and utilise resistors, with a smaller resistance for shorter exposure times.

Automatic exposure devices

These are rarely seen in the veterinary field. These devices allow exposure to occur until chambers under the patient detect a pre-selected exposure. At this point, the exposure will stop. These systems rely on careful positioning and accurate chamber and exposure selection.

Interlocks

Interlocks prevent an exposure being made that can result in over-heating of the target and subsequent damage. A circuit has a number of switches that open and close the circuit. Unless all of the switches are closed, the circuit will not be complete and an exposure will not be possible. Common interlocks include a delay in exposure until the anode rotates correctly ('prep' stage during exposure process), protection from a very high exposure setting and the prevention of movement of a tube suspended from ceiling if there is an obstruction.

Thermal circuit breaker

If the tube and generator overheat, then the circuit will be broken and exposure will be prevented. This happens because the circuit contains a bi-metal strip. The strip will expand if it heats up and the circuit will be broken. The connection will re-form as the strip cools.

Types of X-ray machines

X-ray units fall into a number of distinct categories depending on their generator type, frequency and mobility.

The main categories are mobile, portable or fixed, with the distinction made on the basis of amount of movement possible with each machine. All can be used in veterinary practice. Distinction can also be made on the basis of type of generator used and the frequency of the unit. The choice of X-ray machine in practice will depend on the caseload, the type of examinations expected to be routine and the size and mobility of the unit.

Whichever type of machine is selected, care should be taken to maintain the source–image distance (SID). This is the distance from the point where the X-rays are made on the anode to the image receiver or cassette. This should be constant to prevent problems arising from altering the distance and the impact of the inverse square law.

Fixed X-ray unit

Some tubes may be mounted on the wall, ceiling or floor and are described as fixed units (Figure 5.4). With these machines, care should be taken to keep the tracks or runners clean and free from hair that may impair the movement of the machine. They should also be used with a table of a suitable height with a piece of lead rubber to prevent backscatter under the film. Some units use a cross-track system to allow the unit to cover a large area. The tube support allows movement in the transverse, longitudinal and vertical direction with the X-ray tube supported on a telescopic arm. These movements are usually colour-coded to correspond with the brakes on the tube and the direction of movement.

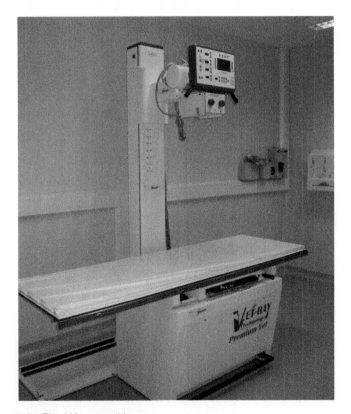

Figure 5.4 Fixed X-ray machine.

Some rooms may have a floor-mounted or table-mounted X-ray tube, which is more cost effective but limits the range of available movement. These units have a track recessed into the floor or attached to the table. This design limits mobility within the imaging room and can also pose a health and safety risk from the collection of hair or fluids.

The alternative arrangement for a fixed unit is to have the X-ray unit fixed to a wall. Whilst ensuring the X-ray machine takes up the minimum amount of space, this arrangement will limit mobility of the machine usually to vertical radiography with the patient positioned close to the supporting wall.

Mobile and portable X-ray units

Mobile and portable units can be used anywhere, with portable units being exactly as the name describes (Figure 5.5). These can be packed away and transported to enable field radiography. This is ideal for equine or farm animal radiography of the extremities, where low-energy machines are able to provide acceptable diagnostic images.

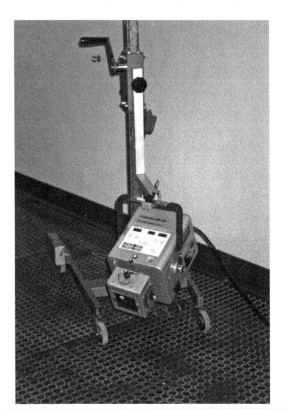

Figure 5.5   Typical design of a digital mobile X-ray unit.

Mobile units are larger than portable units and are able to work at higher exposure levels. They are ideal for a small practice where space is limited and the majority of the work includes small animal extremities, chest and abdomen. Digital mobile units are now available and eliminate the need for cassettes, films, processors or storage space.

Health and safety requirements

- The ceiling should support the weight of the X-ray tube, cables and associated structures.
- Where possible, movement should be automated to prevent physical strain on the operator.
- The X-ray tube should move as freely as the room and mounting system allow.
- Accurate indication of the relationship between the tube, patient, image receiver and table should be visible.
- Utilisation of electromechanical interlocks and counterweight balances to provide a stable and safe piece of equipment.

Power rating

The power rating of an X-ray machine is described in kilowatts. The standard way of calculating this value is to take the maximum mA possible at 100 kV_p for an exposure of 100 milliseconds to give the maximum available power. This may not be accurate if the X-ray unit uses a single-phase waveform, as the current will fluctuate. The calculation of power rating will not give the rating for the X-ray tube, which may be lower.

Further reading

Kings Centre for the Assessment of Radiological Equipment. Available at http://www.kcare.co.uk.

This website provides a whole range of reports and assessments on radiographic equipment.

It is also worth visiting the websites for each of the major equipment manufacturers and suppliers to obtain full details of their equipment.

Revision questions

1 What are the three controls on the X-ray machine control panel?
2 What is the first thing you should check when an X-ray machine is switched on?
3 On the X-ray machine, which control governs the length of time for which the X-rays are produced?

(continued)

4 Which of the following statements about X-ray machines is false?

    a. Portable machines are high-power machines capable of 120 mA.

    b. Some mobile machines are battery-powered.

    c. The control panel can be at some distance from the machine.

    d. Fixed machines can be attached to the ceiling by rails.

5 What does a generator do?

6 Why is rectification useful in radiography?

7 What is a Dose Area Product Meter?

8 What happens in the filament circuit?

9 What units are used for measuring the power rating of an X-ray tube?

10 What is the source–image distance?

Chapter 6

Production of X-rays

Chapter contents

Electron production
Target interactions
X-ray emission spectrum
Altering the emission spectrum
X-ray quantity
X-ray quality
Altering exposure factors
Exposure charts
Further reading

Key points

- X-rays are produced when high-speed projectile electrons collide with the X-ray tube target
- The kinetic energy of projectile electrons gets transferred to target atoms. Approximately 99% of the energy is converted into heat and only about 1% is converted into X-rays
- X-rays are produced from two interactions: bremsstrahlung and characteristic
- X-ray beam quality and quantity are affected by the target material, beam filtration, distance and exposure factors
- Beam filtration affects the beam quality and quantity by removing low-energy X-rays
- The quality of radiation in an X-ray beam is the penetrating ability of the beam
- The quantity of radiation in an X-ray beam is the number of photons in the beam
- kV_p controls the quality of the beam
- mAs affects the quantity of X-rays produced

Practical Veterinary Diagnostic Imaging, Second Edition. Suzanne Easton.
© 2012 John Wiley & Sons, Ltd. Published 2012 by Blackwell Publishing Ltd.

Introduction

The production of X-rays is based on the formation of a current and then the interaction of the electrons in this current with a tungsten target. An mA is applied to the filament at the cathode (negative). This mA heats up the filament and allows electrons to be released. A special focussing cup around the cathode collects and directs the electrons away from the cathode when the potential difference (kV) is applied between the cathode and the target (focal spot) on the tungsten anode (positive). This occurs within a vacuum so that there are no other particles present to interact with the electrons as they pass across to the anode. As the electrons strike the anode, they produce X-rays. Only 1–5% of the energy of the electrons is turned into X-rays; the rest is transformed into heat.

Successful production of X-rays results in the formation of characteristic and brehmsstrahlung radiation. Characteristic radiation has specific properties and interacts with matter in a number of different ways. The interaction depends on the material and the velocity of the X-rays at the time of the interaction.

Electron production

Four conditions are necessary for the production of diagnostic X-rays (Figure 6.1):

1 A source of free electrons.
2 A means to provide the electrons with high kinetic (motion) energy.
3 A method to concentrate the electrons into a beam.
4 A suitable material to rapidly decelerate the electrons.

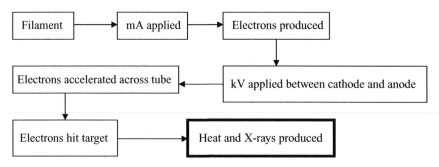

Figure 6.1   Summary of the production of X-rays.

Target interactions

When the high-speed projectile electrons collide with the X-ray tube target, they interact with the orbital electrons or the nuclear field of the target atoms. Kinetic energy transferred from the projectile electrons to the target atoms is converted into heat or X-rays. When projectile electrons strike outer target shell electrons, it puts them in an excited state and, as a result, infrared (heat) radiation is emitted. Approximately 99% of the energy of projectile electrons is converted into heat. Only about 1% of the energy is converted into X-ray photons. Two types of interactions produce X-ray photons: bremsstrahlung interactions and characteristic interactions.

Bremsstrahlung interactions

When an X-ray is first produced, a process called bremsstrahlung occurs as the electron decelerates to produce an X-ray photon. This is sometimes known as braking radiation. As an electron comes near the nucleus of an atom in the target, it will slow down and change its course. During this time, it will lose kinetic energy. This loss in kinetic energy will appear as an X-ray. The X-rays produced in this way can be of different energy levels and the interaction will occur randomly. The energy produced cannot be greater than the kV_p selected. In the diagnostic range, approximately 85% of X-ray emissions are the result of bremsstrahlung interactions (Figure 6.2).

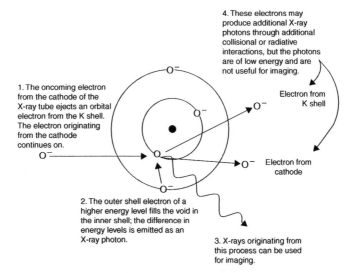

Figure 6.2 Production of bremsstrahlung radiation.

Characteristic interactions

The production of characteristic radiation occurs in a similar way, but the X-rays produced are of a specific energy level. This occurs when the electron from an inner shell is ejected from the atom and an outer shell electron falls into the empty space created. As this outer shell electron moves, an X-ray is emitted. The energy of the X-rays produced will be equal to the energy binding the involved electrons together. Approximately 15% of X-ray emissions are the result of characteristic interactions (Figure 6.3).

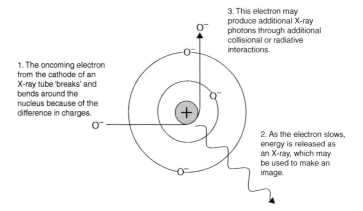

Figure 6.3   Production of characteristic radiation.

X-ray emission spectrum

The X-ray emission spectrum is a demonstration of the energy of each individual X-ray produced during an exposure. In the emission spectrum, the number of X-rays produced is plotted against the energy of each individual X-ray photon. The X-ray spectrum is specific to the type of machine and will alter depending on the type of photon being measured. Changing the kV_p, mA, time and inherent filtration of the machine can alter the spectrum.

Characteristic X-ray spectrum

Characteristic radiation will produce a line spectrum. All of the units will have fixed values that are specific to each individual element. Tungsten will have 15 energy levels. These are demonstrated as straight lines on the emission spectrum, one line for each electron shell of the atom. These are ejected as k or l X-rays depending on the shell that has ejected the electrons and the energy level. These are the thin lines in Figure 6.4. L lines will not be represented if the tube output is demonstrated. This is because the soft (low-energy) radiation will be removed by the aluminium filtration present.

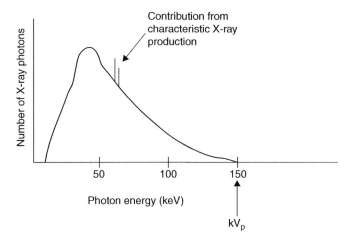

Figure 6.4 Characteristic and bremsstrahlung emission spectrum.

Bremsstrahlung X-ray spectrum

The formation of X-rays through bremsstrahlung will produce a continuous spectrum. This will extend from zero to the maximum energy possessed by the electrons. The majority of X-rays (producing a peak) will have about one-third of the maximum energy. This is the thicker curved line in Figure 6.4.

Altering the emission spectrum

A number of different factors will alter the emission spectrum. If these alterations are understood, then the effects on the resultant image can be understood.

Change in atomic number

The intensity of X-rays produced is directly proportional to the atomic number of the target. If the atomic number is low, then the number of X-rays produced will be lower. The k lines will move to a lower photon energy level. The maximum photon energy and spectrum shape will remain unchanged (Figure 6.5).

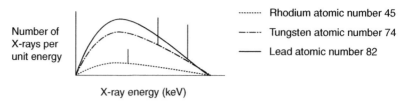

Figure 6.5 The effect of atomic number on emission spectrum.

Change in current (mA)

The mA is directly proportional to the number of X-rays produced. If the mA is doubled, then twice as many electrons will be produced at the cathode, resulting in the production of twice as many X-rays for each energy level. However, the maximum energy levels will remain the same. The k lines will remain at the same energy level (Figure 6.6).

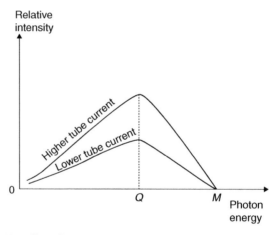

Figure 6.6 The effect of mA on emission spectrum.

Change in kV$_p$

The intensity of X-rays is directly proportional to the square of the kV. If the kV$_p$ is increased, then far more electrons are released from the cathode and so the number of X-rays at each energy level will increase dramatically. This increase will be greater at the higher energy levels. The maximum energy level will also increase. If the kV$_p$ is decreased, the spectral peak will move to a lower value and the k radiation may not be produced (Figure 6.7).

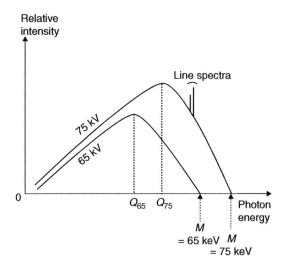

Figure 6.7   The effect of changing the kV_p on emission spectrum.

Increasing the kVp by 15% is equal to doubling the mAs for a given optical density.

Effect of filtration

Alteration in the filtration of the beam will alter the spectral shape. Filtration will remove the low-energy photons from the beam and move the peak to a higher energy level. There will also be a reduction in the intensity, but the maximum photon energy will remain the same (Figure 6.8).

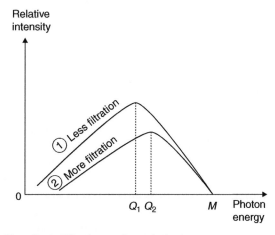

Figure 6.8   The effect of filtration on the emission spectrum.

X-ray quantity

The quantity or the intensity of X-rays produced is the description of the number of X-rays in the useful beam. The useful beam is the beam that forms the radiographic image. The X-ray quantity can be calculated by monitoring the rate of flow of energy through a unit area at right angles to the beam.

The alteration of mAs, kV_p, distance and filtration will all alter the density of the resultant image (optical density). Increasing or decreasing these factors will all increase or decrease the optical density in a similar direction, although the changes may not be of a similar size.

X-ray quality

The X-ray quality describes the penetrating power of the beam. This is measured in terms of the half-value layer, which is the thickness of material that reduces the intensity of the beam to half of its original intensity. This is affected by the kV_p and the filtration used. If the kV is high, the X-rays will penetrate the object being radiographed further than softer, low-energy X-rays. The high-kV X-rays will have a greater half-value layer (Table 6.1).

Table 6.1 Summary of factors affecting X-ray quality and quantity.

Basic factors influencing the quality and quantity of the X-ray beam:

- Target material
- Beam filtration
- Distance
- Prime exposure factors

Altering exposure factors

Source–image distance (SID) or focal film distance (FFD)

SID and FFD are interchangeable terms. The FFD is the distance from the focal spot of the X-ray tube to the film. This distance should be constant during all radiographic examinations, if at all possible. If this distance is altered, the inverse square law can be applied. If the FFD is altered, the number of electrons produced (and therefore X-rays) will also need to be altered to produce a comparable radiograph. The mAs alterations can be calculated as follows:

$$\text{Old mAs} \times \frac{(\text{New distance})^2}{(\text{Old distance})^2} = \text{New mAs}$$

mAs

The mAs is the amperage applied to the tube multiplied by the time that it occurs over. In the ideal situation, the mA should be as high as possible with a short time. This will reduce movement blur from the respiration or movement of the animal. The mAs can be calculated as below. Changes in time or mA can be calculated by rearranging the equation:

$$mAs = mA \times Time(s)$$

kV

Alteration of the kV will alter the penetrating power of the primary beam. If the kV is higher, the mA can be reduced to give a radiograph of similar density. However, this does not mean that the contrast will be similar. From a starting exposure, increasing the kV by 10 will require half the original mAs to give a radiograph of similar density.

60 kV	4 mAs	70 kV	2 mAs
80 kV	1 mAs	90 kV	0.5 mAs

Patient/part thickness

As the size of the part being radiographed increases, so will the kV to allow adequate penetration. In practice, with experience, this calculation will be carried out without measurements being necessary.

Use of grids

Grids reduce the amount of scattered radiation reaching the film, but in so doing, some primary beam or useful beam is absorbed. To compensate for this, the exposure must be increased. The mAs should be multiplied by the grid factor.

Dressings

Wherever possible, dressings should be removed; however, the following acts as a guide:

Fibre glass/vet wrap and bandaging	1.5 × mAs
Plaster of Paris	2 × mAs
Wet plaster of Paris	4 × mAs

Exposure charts

These can be formed within a practice either as a daybook recording all examinations or built up over a period of time for different breeds of animals recorded by region of examination. To make the exposure chart an effective tool, as many factors as possible need to be standardised. As a minimum, this should be the FFD for each examination and the film–screen combination used. The chart can only be used as a guide because each animal and condition will require slightly different exposure factors. The exposure chart is specific to one particular machine, as all tubes will produce slightly different exposure factors, regardless of the settings.

Further reading

Bushong, S. (2004) *Radiologic Science for Technologists: Physics, Biology, and Protection*, 8th edn. St Louis: Elsevier Mosby, pp. 147–160.
This book clearly describes with good diagrams the production of X-rays.
Fauber, T.L. (2004) *Radiographic Imaging and Exposure*, 2nd edn. St Louis: Mosby, pp. 19–32.
This text clearly describes with practical tips the effects of exposure on a radiographic image.

Revision questions

1 Describe the production of bremsstrahlung radiation.

2 Is characteristic radiation produced during a diagnostic examination?

3 Draw a diagram of an emission spectrum.

4 How can the emission spectrum be altered? Give four factors.

5 What percentage change of kV_p is equal to doubling of the mAs?

6 Describe X-ray quantity.

7 What factors can alter the X-ray quantity?

8 What is X-ray quality?

9 How is X-ray quality measured?

10 Give two factors that will alter X-ray quality.

Chapter 7

The Effects of Radiation

Chapter contents

The effect of the X-ray beam striking another atom
Absorption
Attenuation
The effects of ionising radiation on the body
Luminescence
Further reading

Key points

- Classical scattering is a change in the direction of the X-ray photon without a loss in energy
- Compton effect is caused when the incident X-ray photon ionises the atom and the X-ray changes direction and loses energy
- Photoelectric absorption occurs when the X-ray photon is absorbed by one of the electrons in the inner shell of the atom. A photoelectron is emitted with an energy level nearly equal to that of the incident X-ray photon. Characteristic radiation is also emitted as the inner shell fills
- Attenuation is the reduction in the intensity of an X-ray beam as it passes through matter
- Attenuation is the sum of absorption and scatter
- Attenuation in the tissues of the body results in a transfer of energy, and the resulting ionisation may have detrimental effects on the tissue
- X-rays produce fluorescence in phosphors. They are used in intensifying screens

Introduction

As part of the electromagnetic spectrum, X-rays have a number of consistent properties. The key effects of X-rays are:

1 Penetration
2 Absorption

Practical Veterinary Diagnostic Imaging, Second Edition. Suzanne Easton.
© 2012 John Wiley & Sons, Ltd. Published 2012 by Blackwell Publishing Ltd.

3 Biological effects
4 Fluorescence

The effect of the X-ray beam striking another atom

All X-rays interact with matter to produce secondary radiation. Secondary radiation is any radiation produced by an object that has been radiated. This radiation can travel in any direction and is described as scatter. The amount of scattered radiation will depend on the density of the patient and the atomic number of the tissues. If the tissues contain elements with high atomic numbers or the patient is large, scatter will increase. As the size of the field increases, the amount of scatter will increase, so limitation of the primary beam can be used to reduce scattered radiation. As is already known, as the kV_p increases, the wavelength of the primary beam will increase. This will give the primary beam and the secondary radiation more penetrating power and results in more scattered radiation reaching the film. The scattered radiation caused by a patient can be reduced through the use of a grid, discussed later, or the use of a compression band. A compression band will reduce the volume of tissue in a given area and will reduce the necessary exposure. This, in turn, will reduce the kV needed and will increase the contrast of the resultant image. In veterinary work, placing a patient in dorsal or ventral recumbency can reduce the volume of tissue to improve contrast in very large or obese animals. In diagnostic radiography, only the Compton effect and photoelectric absorption will have an effect on the types of scattered radiation produced. The Compton effect will result in no diagnostic information reaching the film and photoelectric absorption results in all the X-ray photons being absorbed. Only X-ray photons that pass through the patient without interacting will produce a diagnostic image.

Classical scattering

Classical scattering is not particularly important in radiography. If the X-ray photon has a low energy level in comparison to the binding energy of the electrons in the matter, it will interact with electrons in the outer shells. This will make the electrons vibrate. The X-ray photon emitted will have the same energy level as the incident photon but will move in a different direction.

Photoelectric absorption

Photoelectric absorption will result in the X-ray photon being totally absorbed by the matter. The X-ray photon interacts with a bound electron as long as the energy of the incoming photon is equal to or greater than the binding energy of the electron. The ejected electron will have kinetic energy that is equal to the binding energy of the incident photon. The ejected electron will travel through matter, losing energy. The atom is left in an excited state. An electron falling from an outer shell into the inner shell, filling the gap fills the vacancy. The energy given off during this movement is emitted as characteristic radiation (Figure 7.1).

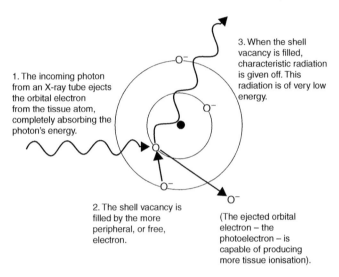

1. The incoming photon from an X-ray tube ejects the orbital electron from the tissue atom, completely absorbing the photon's energy.

3. When the shell vacancy is filled, characteristic radiation is given off. This radiation is of very low energy.

2. The shell vacancy is filled by the more peripheral, or free, electron.

(The ejected orbital electron – the photoelectron – is capable of producing more tissue ionisation).

Figure 7.1 The process of photoelectric absorption.

Photoelectric absorption is more likely to occur in dense tissues or matter containing a high atomic (proton) number. It is also more likely to occur with low-energy X-rays photons.

On an X-ray image, an area with a large number of photoelectric absorption appears white (bone) and areas with lower density, such as air-filled lung tissue, appear black due to the reduction in photoelectric absorption.

Photoelectric absorption plays a part in the following:

1 X-ray tube filtration through the removal of low-energy X-ray using the aluminium filter.
2 The introduction of contrast medium to demonstrate low-density tissue.
3 Shielding through the use of lead that will absorb X-rays due to its density.
4 Radiation dose – lower X-ray exposures will result in more photoelectric absorption interactions within the tissue, increasing the dose to the patient.

Compton effect

The Compton effect will occur when the X-ray photon interacts with a free electron. The energy of the incident photon is shared between the electron and the scattered photon. The photon can be scattered anywhere from $0°$ to $180°$. The electron will always be scattered forward. This is known as the scatter angle. If the scatter angle is small, then the photon has lost energy and the electron has received energy. This type of scattering is not related to atomic number but does depend on the density of electrons present (Figure 7.2).

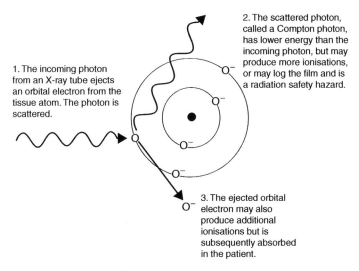

1. The incoming photon from an X-ray tube ejects an orbital electron from the tissue atom. The photon is scattered.

2. The scattered photon, called a Compton photon, has lower energy than the incoming photon, but may produce more ionisations, or may log the film and is a radiation safety hazard.

3. The ejected orbital electron may also produce additional ionisations but is subsequently absorbed in the patient.

Figure 7.2   The Compton effect.

Image degradation caused by Compton scatter

A scattered X-ray photon moving in a forward direction may reach the image receiver.

A forward scattered X-ray photon may leave the body and reach the image receptor. If the X-ray photon has been scattered, it will not travel in a forward direction and will alter the image quality. Scatter will cause what should be 'white' areas on the image to become grey or light grey and thus appear darker. This causes a loss of contrast and degrades the image.

Compton scatter can be reduced by limiting the volume of tissue exposed to the X-ray beam by careful and accurate collimation of the area of interest. Where a large volume must be exposed, such as the abdomen or an equine spine, a radiation grid can be used to absorb, through photoelectric absorption, most of the X-ray photons that have been scattered.

Radiation dose caused by Compton scatter

As most of the scatter occurs in the patients' body, there is no avoiding of interactions of the scatter with other parts of the body. Although such interactions cannot be prevented, they can be reduced through careful and accurate collimation.

Scatter will occur in the X-ray tube but can be prevented from exiting the tube through the design features. The lead within the tube wall will absorb scattered photons, preventing them from exiting the X-ray tube.

The operator can be protected through consistent use of lead screens, doors and protective lead-equivalent aprons.

What happens to the electrons produced?

The photoelectrons and Compton electrons will escape from the atom with kinetic energy. These electrons will interact with neighbouring atoms through ionisation and excitation. This will happen until all the kinetic energy is lost.

A photoelectron or Compton electron will produce several hundred ionisations within a fraction of a millimetre. This process may result in biological effects to the cells.

Absorption

During absorption, the energy from the X-ray photon is transferred to the atoms of the absorber. As more energy is absorbed, the number of X-ray photons passing through the matter and forming the image on the film decreases. This absorption can be as a result of the energy of the X-ray photons or the atomic number of the matter. During absorption, the photoelectric effect will take place (Figure 7.3).

Attenuation

Attenuation is the reduction in intensity of the X-ray beam as it passes through matter. This can be due to absorption or scatter or a combination of both. Every type of matter has a different attenuation coefficient. This is the effectiveness of the matter to attenuate or absorb the radiation passing through. Every X-ray will have a fixed range of attenuation through tissue; this will depend on the atomic

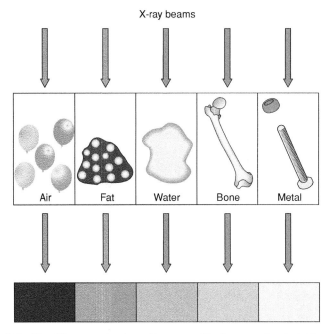

Figure 7.3 The differences in absorption caused by tissue and material type.

number of the atoms involved and the density of the atoms within the tissue. Attenuation is the sum of scattered and absorbed X-ray photons.

Attenuation = Absorption + Scatter

The effects of ionising radiation on the body

Ionising radiation can originate from the X-ray tube or in the form of gamma rays. This radiation damages cells and is not selective of cell type. The effects are more obvious in the immature or rapidly dividing cells. The amount of cell damage is determined by the amount of dose, the type of cell and its maturity. If the cell is still being formed when the dose is received, then the DNA may mutate. Later in the cell cycle, repair may occur.

Biological effects	**Heat, excitation and ionisation**
Cellular effects	**Somatic, carcinogenic and mutation**

Types of effects

Stochastic

This is a genetic effect. There is no safe dose, and as the dose increases, the chance of being affected increases.

Non-stochastic

This type of effect has a threshold level. Below the threshold, the chance of being affected is very low. Once the threshold is reached, the chance of being affected is very high.

Somatic

The person irradiated experiences these effects. Somatic effects will occur during the lifetime of the person. These effects include skin reddening, blood disorders, cataracts or intestinal upset. These changes can happen very soon after exposure.

Genetic

With this type of effect, the effects of the radiation on the genetic make-up of the person may become apparent in future generations. The person receiving the dose will not be affected in their lifetime; however, their future generations may be.

Somatic stochastic

This is a cancer induced by the radiation and will be experienced during a lifetime. The effects may take time before they become evident.

Somatic non-stochastic

This effect of radiation can be used to our advantage in radiotherapy.

Luminescence

Luminescence can be divided into two separate categories: fluorescence and phosphorescence. Both occur when a phosphor is bombarded by radiation; in radiography, the radiation is in the form of X-rays. Fluorescence is the emission of light during exposure, whereas phosphorescence is the afterglow.

Fluorescence occurs when X-ray photons pass through the phosphor layer of the intensifying screen. The phosphor crystal absorbs the X-ray photon. This phosphor becomes excited, emitting ultraviolet and visible light. The visible light is used to make the latent image on a radiographic film.

The phosphor will emit hundreds of light photons for every X-ray photon that strikes it. This is why, along with the fact that radiographic film is more sensitive to light, less exposure is necessary to provide an image if an intensifying screen is used.

Further reading

Harbron, R. (2011) The sunburn effect: deterministic effect of ionising radiation. *Synergy* (February), 22–25.

Harbron, R. (2011) A deadly lottery? Stochastic effects of ionising radiation. *Synergy* (March), 26–29.

Harbron, R. (2011) X-ray energy and its effect on image formation using kV_p to best effect. *Synergy* (May), 22–27.

Harbron, R. (2011) Illuminating the shadows: scattering in radiation. *Synergy* (June), 16–19.

This is a series of articles that discuss ionising radiation and its effects. They provide valuable information to radiographers.

Revision questions

1 Describe the Compton effect.

2 Describe photoelectric absorption.

3 What is the relationship between the density of a material and the absorption of X-rays?

4 What is attenuation?

5 What is attenuation equal to?

6 Describe why scattered radiation can be a hazard.

7 Which tissue type results in the highest photoelectric absorption?

8 How can Compton scatter be minimised?

9 What is a stochastic effect of ionising radiation?

10 Where is fluorescence used?

Chapter 8

Control of the Primary Beam and Scatter

Chapter contents

Light beam diaphragm
Factors affecting scattered radiation
Function of grids
Construction of a grid
Types of grid
Choosing a grid
Problems with using a grid
Air gap technique
Further reading

Key points

- Collimators can limit the primary beam
- Radiation safety is improved by limiting the primary beam
- Light beam diaphragm collimators give most accurate limitation of the primary beam
- Light beam diaphragm has lead leaves with bevelled edges
- Scattered radiation is dependent on patient size and the kV used
- Grids absorb unwanted secondary radiation
- A grid is made up of lead strips spaced with a radiolucent material
- The lead strips absorb the scatter
- The grid ratio is the height of the strips to the width of the spaces
- Grids can be either parallel, focussed, pseudo-focussed or cross-hatched
- To eliminate grid lines, the grid can be moved
- Care must be taken with grids to ensure that manufacturer guidelines are followed
- The grid should be flat and in the correct orientation to the tube when used
- The air gap technique can also remove scatter

Practical Veterinary Diagnostic Imaging, Second Edition. Suzanne Easton.
© 2012 John Wiley & Sons, Ltd. Published 2012 by Blackwell Publishing Ltd.

Introduction

Control of the primary beam is important in the maintenance of high radiation safety standards. If the primary beam is not limited, there will be increased levels of scattered radiation produced, leading to an increased risk of exposure to the radiographer. Collimation in whatever form will also improve the visual quality of the resultant image.

Light beam diaphragm

This is an aluminium box that is lead-lined, fixed below the port on the tube. The bottom of the box has a Perspex window. Just above the Perspex window, there are two pairs of adjustable lead leaves. The opposing faces are bevelled at 45° to give total closure (Figure 8.1).

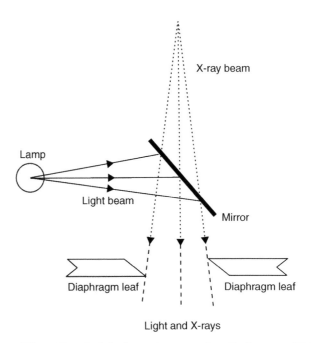

Figure 8.1 Effect of bevelled diaphragm leaves on the effectiveness of limitation of the primary beam.

A light is displayed at the same angle as the primary beam through the use of a series of mirrors. The mirrors do not alter the beam. The unit has an automatic timer so that it switches off after a set period of time, therefore preventing it from overheating. The diaphragm box should rotate to give flexibility on patient position and collimation.

Beam-centring devices

These devices allow control of the alignment of the tube with the patient and the area of irradiation to the patient. They are usually built into the Perspex window on the bottom of the light beam diaphragm. The Perspex has a cross marking the centre of the focal spot, and light will demonstrate the edges of the collimated field. In older machines, the centring device may need to be removed before the exposure is made as it may show on the radiograph.

Factors affecting scattered radiation

Secondary radiation is any radiation other than the primary beam. Any object that has been irradiated can produce secondary radiation. If this secondary radiation is in any direction other than that of the primary beam, it is known as scatter. This can also be in the form of backscatter from the table or the cassette.

Patient size

If the patient is large, their overall volume will be greater, and this will increase the amount of scatter generated. This can be reduced through the use of a compression band that will reduce the volume of tissue in any one place at a given time. This in turn will reduce the scatter produced and increase the contrast of the resultant image.

Kilovoltage

The voltage selected for an examination will alter the amount of scatter produced. As the wavelength of the primary beam increases with an increase in kilovoltage, so is the amount of scatter reaching the film. The amount of Compton scatter will increase as the kV increases.

Function of grids

The grid has two functions:

1 The grid absorbs secondary scattered radiation that may have a detrimental effect on the final image.
2 The grid allows the primary beam to pass through unaffected to form the useful image on the film.

Construction of a grid

The grid is usually seen as a sheet of metal from the outside, but its internal structure is made up of two very distinct parts: the lead strips and radiolucent spaces. The outside of the grid is made of aluminium, as it is strong and gives high precision. The aluminium casing also prevents moisture entering the grid and gives it rigidity (Figure 8.2).

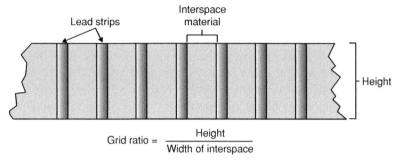

$$\text{Grid ratio} = \frac{\text{Height}}{\text{Width of interspace}}$$

Figure 8.2   The construction of a parallel anti-scatter grid.

Lead strips

The lead strips absorb the scattered radiation that does not pass through the radiolucent spacers. The lead absorbs the lower energy scattered radiation as it has a high atomic number and a high mass density. Lead is used because it is cheap and fairly easy to shape. In any type of grid, there will be a maximum of 40 strips of lead in every centimetre of grid.

Radiolucent interspace

This is made of plastic, aluminium or carbon fibre. The material used must be rigid to maintain the position of the lead strips. The interspace will allow the primary beam to pass straight through whilst filtering the scattered radiation. Despite the primary beam passing straight through the interspace, some of the primary beam will be absorbed by the lead strips and so a higher exposure will be necessary when using a grid (Figure 8.3).

Grid ratio

The grid ratio is the height of the strips to the width of the interspace. If the ratio is high, more scattered radiation will be absorbed. If a grid has a high ratio, then a higher exposure must be used to compensate

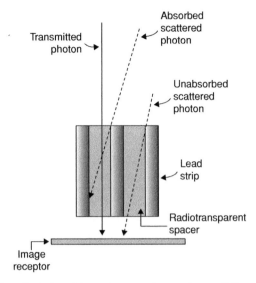

Figure 8.3   The effect of a grid on primary and secondary radiation.

for the increase in absorption of the primary beam. Ratios range from 3:1 to 16:1, although the ratio that is commonly used is 6:1.

4:1	**A ratio of 4:1 means that the height of the lead strips is 4 times the width of the spacer.**
10:1	**A ratio of 10:1 means that the height of the lead strips is 10 times the width of the spacer.**

Grid lattice

The grid lattice describes the lines per centimetre. This is the number of strips to each centimetre. As the number of lines increases, both the exposure needed to produce a diagnostic radiograph and the amount of scatter absorbed increase.

Grid factor

When a grid is used, the amount of exposure required increases. The exposure factor increased is the mAs. The amount of exposure increase can be calculated. Depending on the type of grid used, the grid factor is usually about 4, but will depend on the grid ratio.

$$\text{Grid factor} = \frac{\text{Exposure with the grid}}{\text{Exposure without the grid}}$$

Types of grid

Parallel

A parallel grid has lead strips that are vertical and parallel to each other. This type of grid is the most simple to use, as it does not have to be used with a specific focal film distance or specific centring point. The tube can be angled so long as it is parallel to the lead strips. This type of grid is also the cheapest to buy. Some cut-off of radiation will occur on the edges of the film because of the divergence of the primary beam (Figure 8.4).

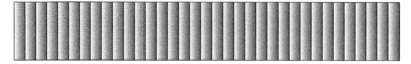

Figure 8.4   Parallel grid.

Focussed

With this type of grid, the lead strips and interspacers are titled with an increasing angle further from the centre of the grid. This allows for the diverging primary beam on the edges of the useful beam to pass through the grid. If the lead strips were extended, they would meet at a point in front of the grid. This is known as the grid focus and this is where the tube should be positioned to get the maximum performance from the grid. Centring and focus-to-grid distance need to be accurate, otherwise cut-off will occur. If the grid is used back to front, cut-off will occur (Figure 8.5).

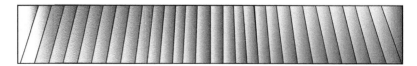

Figure 8.5   Focussed grid.

Psuedo-focussed grid

With this type of grid, the lead slats are parallel but tapered. This means that the diverging beam is able to pass through the grid without being absorbed, as it is in a parallel grid.

Cross-hatched parallel grid

> This type of grid has parallel lead strips laid at 90° to each other. This gives excellent removal of scatter but does require a large increase in exposure. The positioning with this type of grid needs to be accurate.

Moving grids (Potter–Bucky grid)

> The use of a stationary grid will produce an image with very fine lines from the lead strips. To eliminate this effect, the grid can be moved very rapidly to blur out the lines. This type of grid is usually parallel with the grid mounted beneath the tabletop. When the exposure is made, the grid moves rapidly from side to side; on termination of the exposure, the grid will stop moving. This movement must be smooth and uninterrupted.

Choosing a grid

> The choice of a grid will depend on the funds available at the time of choice and the type of work that it will be used for. A parallel grid is good for day-to-day veterinary work, but if funding allows, a pseudo-focussed grid is the grid of choice. Cross-hatched parallel grids should be used if a large amount of farm animal or equine work is to be carried out.
>
> A grid should be used when X-raying any patient or part of patient over 10 cm thick. Below this level, scatter will not be of a level to influence the image quality.

Problems with using a grid

> Grids should be used with care, otherwise a number of problems might occur. If a grid is dropped, then bending of the lead strips is a possibility, which will have a detrimental effect on the function of the grid. The recommendations of the manufacturer should be followed at all time for the best results from the grid. This includes using the correct focal distance and using the grid the correct way round (grids have a back and a front) with the tube side facing the tube. If the grid is used back to front, the primary beam will be absorbed on the edges and will only pass directly through the middle of the film. This will give an image with cut-off, where the middle is adequately exposed, but the edges will have varying densities. This can also happen with incorrect centring or tilting of the grid or use of wrong focus-to-grid distance.

Air gap technique

If the exposure cannot be safely increased when using a grid with a large patient, then the air gap technique can be used. This is an ideal technique for imaging the equine chest or spine. A gap is left between the patient and the film. The gap will allow the scatter produced in the body to be absorbed by the air due to the inverse square law. The scatter is of a lower energy. As the distance will increase, the scatter will have a lower energy level and less of an effect on the film. The scattered radiation can also be lost through divergence after exiting the patient. The air gap should be a minimum of 15 cm, up to a maximum of 300 cm (Figure 8.6).

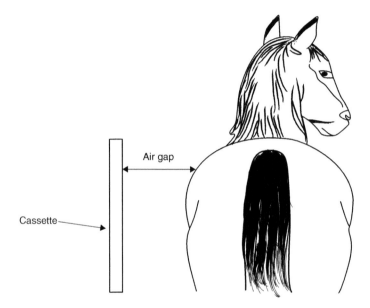

Figure 8.6 Air gap technique.

Further reading

Fauber, T.L. (2008) *Radiographic Imaging and Exposure*, 3rd edn. St Louis: Mosby.
This book contains a lot of useful information on the use of grids and the effect on image quality.

Revision questions

1 Which of the following statements are incorrect when discussing collimation?

  a. The area exposed should never be larger than the film size used.

(continued)

    b. The useful beam should be limited to the smallest area practicable and consistent with the objectives of the examination.

    c. The beam should be collimated to the area of the largest cassette in general use.

2 Give two ways of controlling the primary beam once it has left the X-ray tube.

3 Why are the edges of the lead leaves in a collimator bevelled?

4 How does patient size affect the amount of scatter produced?

5 Describe the construction of a grid.

6 What is the grid factor?

7 How are focussed and pseudo-focussed grids different?

8 What size of patient or patient part is suitable for using a grid to improve the image?

9 What is the air gap technique?

10 What should be a minimum size of the air gap for it to be effective?

Chapter 9

Radiographic Film

Chapter contents

Film construction
Types of film
Formation of the latent image
Care and storage of films
Film sensitivity
Further reading

Key points

- Film is made up of distinct layers
- The base is made of polyester and supports the emulsion
- The subbing layer is composed of gelatine and forms an adhesive for the emulsion
- The emulsion is made up of gelatine, with silver halide grains in suspension
- The gelatine prevents the silver halide grains from bunching
- Grains of silver halide may be globular or tabular
- Emulsion can be sensitised, using dyes, to different wavelengths of light
- The supercoat is a very thin layer of gelatine that will protect the film during processing and storage
- In single-sided films, an anti-halation layer and curl layer are placed on the reverse of the base
- Screen film is designed to be used in conjunction with intensifying screens
- Duplitised film has emulsion on both sides and is used with two screens
- Non-screen film is exposed using X-rays alone
- Non-screen film requires between 5 and 25 times more exposure than screen film
- Radiation-monitoring film is duplitised but has emulsions of different speeds

---

Practical Veterinary Diagnostic Imaging, Second Edition. Suzanne Easton.
© 2012 John Wiley & Sons, Ltd. Published 2012 by Blackwell Publishing Ltd.

- Polaroid film can be used where no processing facilities are available
- Films should be stored upright in a dry, cool room with good ventilation
- Film boxes should not be stacked as the film is sensitive to pressure
- Film should be used in date order
- The latent image is formed through the interaction of light with the silver halide crystals in the emulsion
- Film sensitivity is sometimes described as the speed of a film
- A film with a high speed will require less exposure than a slower film to produce an image of a similar density
- Film duplication uses a special film that works in reverse to a conventional film

Introduction

The production of a radiograph relies upon the exposure of a patient to radiation and the formation of a latent image either on a radiographic film that can be viewed at a later date or, more recently, in the form of a digital image. This chapter examines the 'make-up' of a radiographic film and the formation of a latent image that forms the permanent image during development.

Film construction

Radiographic film is made up of a number of distinct layers, all with specific functions. Whether a film is duplitised (two emulsion sides) or is single-sided, it will have a base layer, a subbing layer, an emulsion and a supercoat to protect the emulsion. If the film is duplitised, the layers will be duplicated on the reverse side of the base. If the film is single-sided, it will have an anti-halation layer and an anti-curl layer on the reverse side of the base (Figure 9.1).

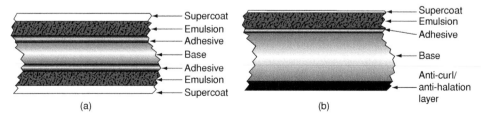

Figure 9.1   Cross-section through (a) duplitised and (b) single-sided emulsion film.

Film base

The film base provides a support for the emulsion and is usually transparent to transmitted light when the radiograph is being reviewed. Polyester is usually the chosen compound, as it is strong, flexible and chemically inert. It maintains its shape and form despite changes in moisture and temperature. Polyester can be produced of a uniform thickness so that an even coating of the emulsion is possible. This is essential, as varying thickness of emulsion will result in an uneven image. The base usually has a blue dye added during manufacturing, and this colour will remain consistent from one batch to another. The film base is usually 0.18 mm thick.

Subbing layer

The subbing layer is composed of gelatine and reactive ester salts. This layer forms an adhesive for the emulsion. If the subbing layer is not used, the emulsion will peel away from the base when it is dry and form a layer of sludge when it is wet. Some manufacturers add a dye to prevent crossover from occurring.

> **Crossover occurs when light passes from one screen, through the film, and exposes the opposing side of the film. This light travels a larger distance than normal and will result in greater divergence and unsharpness.**

Emulsion

The emulsion contains the active part of the film. The emulsion is made up of gelatine, with small crystals of silver halides suspended throughout. Gelatine is used as it can exist as a liquid or a solid and can be applied to the film base easily and evenly as a liquid and can then become a solid suitable for storage and use. The gelatine is permeable to water and will allow the processing chemicals access to the silver halide crystals. The gelatine will also keep the silver halide grains separated to prevent clumping and their uneven distribution. The silver halide grains may be either tabular or globular. The globular grains are monochromatic (sensitive to blue light); tabular grains are orthochromatic or sensitive to blue and green lights. The tabular grains are of a particular shape, which depends on their manufacture, and will fit closely together, giving increased resolution, less crossover and a greater light absorption. Grain size and shape will also enhance the image quality due to changes in the amount of unsharpness caused by the grains (Figure 9.2).

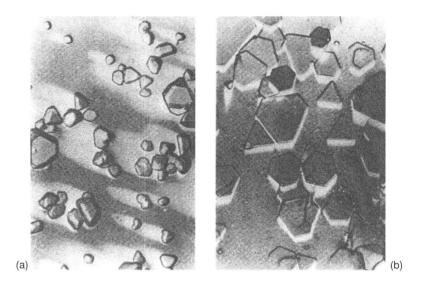

Figure 9.2   Film coverage of (a) globular and (b) tabular grains.

Some emulsions will be sensitised to prevent certain colours of light from passing through. The silver halide is manufactured within the gelatine, following a reaction of silver nitrate and a halide compound. This technique is used to ensure that the silver halide is not exposed to any radiation prior to use. If the film is duplitised, the emulsion will be applied to both sides of the base. If the film is single-sided, only one emulsion layer will be added to the base. In single-sided and direct exposure films, the emulsion will be thicker than that found on duplitised film.

Supercoat

The supercoat is a very thin layer of gelatine that will protect the film during processing and during handling after processing. The surface is semi-matt to help the rollers in the processor move the film.

Anti-halation/curl layer

This layer is found in single-sided film. As the film is processed, the emulsion swells, and this causes the base to curl. In duplitised film, the two emulsion layers will counteract each other. In single-sided films, the second side is coated with a layer of gelatine to prevent the film from curling.

A dye is also added to the backing to prevent scattered light reflected from the base of the film influencing the true image. This reflection is known as halation. The colour of this dye will vary depending on the colour sensitivity of the film (Figure 9.3).

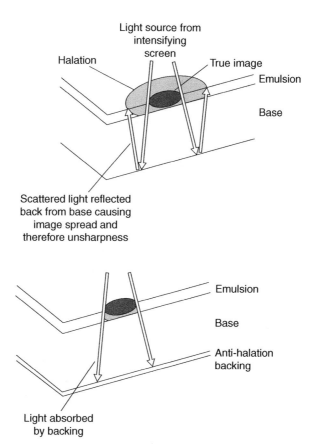

Figure 9.3   Effect of an anti-halation layer.

Types of film

Screen film

Screen film is designed to be used in conjunction with intensifying screens. The image on the film will be formed through direct exposure to X-rays but mainly through light emitted from the phosphors on the screens. The use of two screens will double the efficiency of the X-ray beam and reduce the exposure required.

There are two main types of radiographic film in use: duplitised and single-sided. Duplitised film has two emulsions that reduce the number of X-rays necessary to produce a diagnostic image. These will lessen the wear on the X-ray tube and will increase the contrast on the film. Single-sided screen film has one emulsion layer that reduces crossover and parallax, giving a more detailed image. This increased detail is at the cost of a reduction of exposure and image contrast.

Non-screen film

This type of film relies on direct exposure to produce an image. It is used in human dental radiography and mainly in intra-oral examinations of the nasal chambers in the veterinary field. The emulsion layer is thicker so that more silver halide crystals are present to form the latent image. Non-screen film gives greater detail but requires a much higher exposure (typically, 5–25 times the exposure necessary for normal screen radiography). Larger non-screen films suitable for intra-oral examinations are difficult to obtain and so single-sided film cut to size and placed in a light tight envelope can be used. Due to the thickened emulsion and enlarged grain size, this type of film will require longer processing times than screen film.

Radiation-monitoring film

This type of film is similar to non-screen film in appearance. Although it is duplitised, it has different speeds of emulsion ion each side. This ensures that a wide range of exposure levels can be recorded and monitored. If a large exposure is received, the whole film may become black with a fast emulsion, but this can be removed to demonstrate the density of the slower emulsion giving an accurate estimation of the dose received.

Formation of the latent image

The formation of a latent image is a series of steps involving the interaction of light or X-rays with a silver halide crystal. The silver and bromine atoms are fixed in a lattice. Each crystal is charged as silver loses an electron to form a bond with bromine. The atom is not rigid and so the silver ions will be found within the crystal, whilst the negatively charged bromine atoms will be found on the surface of the crystal.

Silver halide reaction

The interaction of light or X-rays with the crystal will result in the release of electrons. The electrons will migrate to the sensitivity speck within the crystal. This will allow the formation of metallic silver at the sensitivity speck with negative bromine atoms being released. The will be repeated every time the crystal is exposed to light. Eventually, the negative surface charge of bromine will disappear and the amount of silver in the crystal will increase. This collection of silver atoms is the latent image. The remaining silver halide will be converted during processing to a visible image (Figure 9.4).

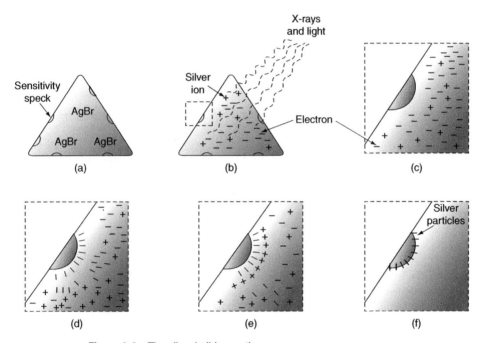

Figure 9.4 The silver halide reaction.

Care and storage of films

Film is sensitive to light, radiation and moisture, and so it needs to be stored to prevent damage from any of these factors. The film is well packaged by the manufacturers and should be kept in this packaging until ready for use.

Expiry dates and stock rotation

A careful note of the expiry date should be made and older stock should be used first. Storage of film is not ideal over longer periods of time and so small regular orders of film mean that it will be in better condition when it is needed.

Protection of the film

Under pressure or when handled roughly, the emulsion can be damaged and artefacts will be seen on the resultant image. Films should be stored vertically to prevent the pressure from other boxes damaging the film.

The film is also sensitive to dampness and moisture and so the room used for its storage should be dry and cool with good ventilation. If the room temperature drops below 15°C, then the box should be brought back to room temperature slowly before use.

Care should be taken to avoid storing the film in the same room as the X-ray equipment or next door to the X-ray room if a horizontal beam is used. Any exposure to radiation will result in fogging of the film.

The film should also be stored away from certain chemicals and fumes, especially those found in the processing chemistry.

Storage of opened boxes

Once opened, boxes of films should be stored in either a specially designed film hopper or in a light-tight drawer. The film should remain in the boxes with the internal wrappings folded over and the lid securely on.

Film sensitivity

It is already known that X-ray film is more sensitive to the light from intensifying screen than X-rays alone. Light is made up of different colours, and the emulsion will react differently to the component colours of light. This response can be controlled by the addition of dyes during manufacture. Without a sensitiser, the emulsion is more sensitive to blue, violet and ultraviolet lights. This type of emulsion is known as monochromatic film. If the sensitiser is present, then the range of colour sensitivity can be increased to include green light. This film is known as orthochromatic. Some film sensitivity can be increased to include red light. This type of film is described as panchromatic.

A graph can be plotted to demonstrate the sensitivity of the film (speed) against the wavelength of light that it is exposed to.

Film speed	*The sensitivity of film to light or radiation*
	Fast films require less exposure to give a similar film when using a slow film.

Sensitivity is calculated and assessed by measurement of the densities produced when a film is subjected to different wavelengths of light for equal exposure times. This curve will determine the film–screen combination possible and the type of safelight needed in the darkroom to protect the film from exposure. Peak sensitivity is always shown as 1 (Figure 9.5).

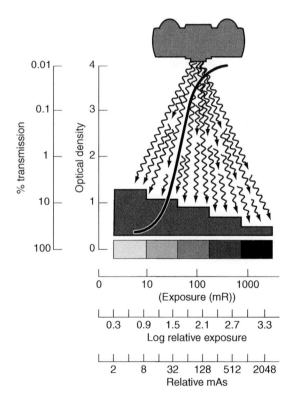

Figure 9.5   Sensitivity curve of a common orthochromatic film.

Further reading

Ball, J., Price, T. (1998) *Chesneys' Radiographic Imaging*, 6th edn. Oxford: Blackwell Science.
This provides a clear explanation of all aspects of films and processing.

Revision questions

1 Draw a diagram of a duplitised film.

2 What are the structural differences between duplitised and single-sided film?

3 Why is gelatine used as the support for the silver halide crystals in the emulsion?

4 How is the emulsion of a film sensitised?

5 What is halation?

6 Why should an animal be anaesthetised when using a non-screen film?

7 What other types of film are available beyond conventional duplitised film?

8 How should radiographic film be stored?

9 Outline the four stages of the silver halide reaction.

10 What is film speed?

Chapter 10

Intensifying Screens and Cassettes

Chapter contents

The construction of intensifying screens
Film–screen combinations
Film–screen contact
Care of intensifying screens
Construction of cassettes
Care and use of cassettes
Further reading

Key points

- An intensifying screen converts X-rays into light
- An intensifying screen reduces the patient dose
- Intensifying screens are composed of a layer of phosphor crystals in a binder
- The phosphor layer is covered in a protective coating
- The main categories of intensifying screens are either rare earth or fast tungstate
- The intensification factor is the exposure required to produce a satisfactory image using intensifying screens
- Screens have three speeds: slow, medium and fast
- The faster an intensifying screen, the lower the exposure necessary to produce a diagnostic image
- Film–screen contact must be good to prevent a loss in detail
- Screens must be protected from scratches, chemical splashes and moisture
- Cassettes contain the film and screens
- The cassette maintains good film–screen contact and prevents light from reaching the film
- The cassette is usually made of plastic or carbon fibre
- The cassette should have low beam absorption

Practical Veterinary Diagnostic Imaging, Second Edition. Suzanne Easton.
© 2012 John Wiley & Sons, Ltd. Published 2012 by Blackwell Publishing Ltd.

Introduction

Intensifying screens are found within the cassette used for radiographic examinations. The screen converts the energy from the X-ray beam into light and this light exposes the film. This reduces the exposure necessary to produce a diagnostic radiograph and, at the same time, improves radiation safety. Less than 1% of the X-ray beam actually exposes the radiographic film; the remainder of the exposure coming from the light emitted from intensifying screens.

The construction of intensifying screens

Intensifying screens are constructed in sizes corresponding to the cassette size. Radiographic film is sandwiched between a pair of intensifying screens inside the cassette. If two screens are to be used, double-emulsion film is used. If more detail is required, a single screen can be used. If a single screen is to be used, a single-emulsion film will be necessary. The emulsion side of the film should be in contact with the intensifying screen.

The screen is composed of four distinct parts: the protective coating, phosphor layer, reflective layer and the base (Figure 10.1).

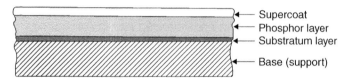

— Supercoat
— Phosphor layer
— Substratum layer
— Base (support)

Figure 10.1   Cross-sectional view of an intensifying screen.

Protective coating

The outer layer of the intensifying screen is the protective coating made from acetate. This is the part of the screen in contact with the X-ray film. It will protect the screen against abrasions, moisture and staining. The coating will also reduce static electricity that may cause an artefact. The protective coating can undergo routine cleaning without any damage if strict guidelines are followed. This layer extends around the back of the screen where it provides a non-curl backing.

Reflective layer

The reflective layer is made of either magnesium oxide or titanium dioxide. This layer will redirect light emitted in a direction that will not expose the film. This will increase the function of the intensifying screen. Some intensifying screens may contain dyes that will absorb this stray light. This will prevent image blur, but will not improve the function of the intensifying screen.

Base

The base is at the back of the intensifying screen. It acts as a support for the screen. It is made of either high-grade cardboard or polyester. These materials are usually chosen for their strong moisture-resistant property whilst remaining flexible. The base must also not react with the phosphor layer or be visible on the resultant image.

Fluorescent phosphor layer

This is the layer within the intensifying screen that is active. It contains a layer of tiny phosphor crystals suspended in a binder of polyurethane. The binder holds the crystals together and prevents moisture affecting them. The binder also contains a coloured pigment or carbon granules that function in a similar way as the dye in the reflective layer. The combination and proportion of these components will determine the speed of the intensifying screen.

The phosphors selected must be very good at absorbing X-rays and must fluoresce well with some afterglow. This afterglow is not used in radiography and will not be described any further. The two main types of phosphors used are either from the rare earth group or calcium tungstate. Rare earth intensifying screens are more effective than calcium tungstate at changing X-ray photons to light (15–20% efficiency compared to 3–5% efficiency with calcium tungstate). Some rare earth screens will have an impurity added to alter the colour of light emitted and the intensity of the light. The rare earth screens contain oxysulphides of gadolinium, lanthanum, yttrium or any of the other elements from the rare earth group of the periodic table. Calcium tungstate was the original phosphor used for radiography and emits blue light.

Film–screen combinations

To ensure that the best is made of the screens and the film available, a number of factors need to be considered.

Light emission and film selection

The colour emitted from the screen needs to be matched with the colour sensitivity of the film. If the screen phosphor emits green light, then it should be used with orthochromatic film. This ensures that the point of maximum sensitivity of the film matches the maximum light emission from the screen. This means that the optimum speed for the system is obtained. If the film sensitivity is not matched to the light emitted from the screens, then the effects of using the intensifying screen will be reduced (Table 10.1).

Table 10.1   Film–screen combinations.

Phosphor type	Colour emitted from screen	Colour sensitivity of film
Calcium tungstate	Blue	Blue (monochromatic)
Rare earth	Green (sometimes blue)	Blue or green (orthochromatic)

Speed

Intensifying screens are usually divided into three categories: slow, medium and fast. The distinction between the categories will depend on the intensification factor or the exposure required to produce a suitable, diagnostic image using intensifying screens. The screens usually come in pairs of similar speeds, although the screen placed on the back of the cassette will have a thicker layer of phosphors. This ensures that the film is evenly exposed. Uneven exposure may occur, as the X-rays reaching the second screen will have passed through the film and front screen, losing energy on the way. This may reduce the light emitted from each phosphor, reducing the exposure to the film.

The speed of screen can be altered by the phosphor grain size, the thickness of the intensifying layer, the presence or absence of a reflective layer and the amount of crossover that may occur from screen to film (Table 10.2).

Table 10.2   Screen speeds.

Screen	Speed	Uses
High resolution	Slow	Fine detail, needs higher exposure; so should be used where lower exposure factors are acceptable
Regular	Medium	General radiography
Fast	Fast	Produces a darker radiographic image for given exposure factors when compared to regular or high-resolution screens Ideal for use where movement may be a problem

Single-screen use

A single screen can be used with specifically produced films. The screen is placed at the back of the cassette to prevent unnecessary divergence of the light prior to reaching the film emulsion. This will improve the sharpness of the resultant image. This type of screen will improve image quality and sharpness, but will require a high exposure to produce a diagnostic image.

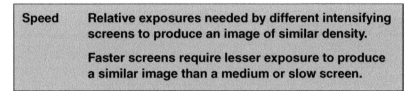

Speed	Relative exposures needed by different intensifying screens to produce an image of similar density.
	Faster screens require lesser exposure to produce a similar image than a medium or slow screen.

Assessing the speed of a new film–screen combination

Every intensifying screen and film combination will require specific exposure factors. If a new set of screens or film is used, the change in speed can be assessed by imaging either a step wedge or a specimen using both combinations (new and old). This will demonstrate the changes necessary in exposure factor to produce a similar radiographic density (Figure 10.2).

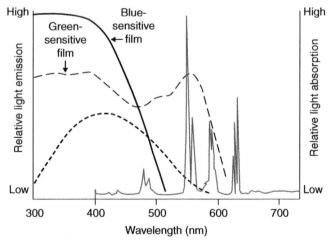

Figure 10.2 Diagram showing emission and absorption spectra for rare earth and calcium tungstate intensifying screens.

Quantum mottle

If a very fast film–screen combination is used with low exposure factors, quantum mottle may occur. This appears as a mottled or even spotty appearance in the resultant image. This occurs if there are not enough photons of light to produce an image on the film. This may be due to the inability of the film to detect the small amount of light or the lack of light produced in the first instance from the intensifying screens.

Film–screen contact

Contact between the screens and film is essential if a high-quality or sharp radiograph is to be obtained. If the contact between the film and screens is not even, areas of the radiograph will appear blurred and unsharp. This effect will occur as the light has spread out through divergence before coming into contact with the film emulsion. Divergence from a number of phosphor crystals may overlap to increase the unsharpness further. Poor film–screen contact can be assessed by placing a wire mesh (metal strip with sequins removed is adequate) on top of the cassette and producing a radiograph. If the there is poor contact, the edges of the circles will be fuzzy and not sharp.

Care of intensifying screens

Any intensifying screen that is damaged cannot be repaired and is useless for the intended function. If one screen gets damaged, it is usually necessary to replace both screens. The function of the screen can be impaired by dust, foreign matter such as animal hair, finger marks or stains. Care should be taken not to touch the screens unnecessarily or leave the cassettes open longer than is necessary as this increases the chances of spillage occurring or something being dropped directly onto the screen. The screens are very sensitive to moisture and temperature, so careful consideration should be given to their storage.

Cleaning screens

Screens should be cleaned regularly to remove any dust or other foreign material from their surfaces. This can be done easily using a mild liquid detergent or a proprietary screen cleaner:

- A soft cloth, but not cotton wool (as it leaves tiny fibres), should be moistened with the detergent and wiped gently over the screen.
- The screen should never become wet, and spillage on the back of the screen must be avoided.

- The screen should then be wiped clean using a fresh, dry cloth or a piece of gauze.
- The cassette should then be left standing upright and slightly open to allow it to dry.
- It is a good idea to record when this is done.

Construction of cassettes

The screens and film of choice are contained within a cassette. This will protect them from damage and prevent dust accumulation on the screens. The cassette will also maintain close contact between the film and screens and also prevent light reaching the film and causing fogging. The insides of all cassettes are black to prevent the reflection of internal light.

Cassette front

The front of the cassette is of a uniform thickness and should conform to British Standards (BS 4304/1968). If the cassette is made of plastic, it should have an aluminium equivalent of no more than 0.2 mm. This will minimise the attenuation of the beam. The front is usually made from plastic or carbon fibre. This provides stiffness whilst still being lightweight. The materials used will also have a low absorption of the beam. Carbon fibre will reduce patient dose especially at lower kilovoltage levels. The front of the cassette will also incorporate a recessed well that will contain the screen and a lead strip to block radiation. This allows for patient identification.

Cassette back

The cassette back is usually of a similar material to the front and is lined with lead foil to protect the film from backscatter. The back is usually curved to ensure good film–screen contact. It may also contain a foam pressure pad under the intensifying screen to increase film–screen contact further.

Closure

All cassettes have a method of ensuring that the cassette remains closed and that adequate film–screen contact is maintained. These methods range from spring clips made of metal to plastic locking bars and plastic clips.

Care and use of cassettes

Cassettes can be damaged and, therefore, care should be taken:

- Use them gently.
- Do not drop them.
- Carry a few at a time.
- Cassettes can be damaged if they are stored at an angle; so they should be as near to vertical as possible.
- If the cassette is used under a patient, the use of a cassette tunnel should be considered to prevent unnecessary pressure being applied to the cassette.
- Try to avoid getting the cassettes wet. If unavoidable, cover the cassette in a waterproof covering (carrier bag is adequate!).
- Number all cassettes, and keep a record of their first use, any damage that occurs and any maintenance that is carried out.

Further reading

Ball, J., Price, T. (1998) *Chesneys' Radiographic Imaging*, 6th edn. Oxford: Blackwell Science.
This provides a clear explanation of all aspects of films and processing.

Revision questions

1 Describe the function of an intensifying screen.

2 How does a phosphor grain convert X-rays into light?

3 Name the three speeds of a screen and when each may be used.

4 What are the two main types of phosphor used in an intensifying screen?

5 Give two factors that can alter the speed of a screen.

6 Why is film–screen contact so essential?

7 How would you clean a screen?

8 Describe the layers within an X-ray cassette.

9 Why are the insides of a cassette black?

10 Give three main points to consider when caring for a cassette.

Chapter 11

Processing the Radiographic Film

Chapter contents

The stages of processing
Developer
Fixer
Parts of the automatic processor
Replenishment
Silver recovery
The darkroom
Control of substances hazardous to health (COSHH)
   regulations
Other methods of processing
Further reading

Key points

- There are four main stages of processing: development, fixing, washing and drying
- Development converts the latent image to a visible image
- Exposed silver halides are reduced to metallic silver
- Sensitivity speck allows developer solution to penetrate the grain
- Fixer stops the development process
- Fixer clears the image by removing silver halide crystals from the emulsion
- Automatic processors rely on a film transportation system to take the film from one tank to the next
- Squeegee rollers remove excess chemistry between tanks
- The time the film spends in each tank is altered by the depth of the tank
- Water is used to maintain the temperature of an automatic processor
- Algae should not be allowed to build up in the wash tanks as they cause artefacts on the radiographic image
- Films are dried using an electric heater or infrared lamps surrounded by blowers

Practical Veterinary Diagnostic Imaging, Second Edition. Suzanne Easton.
© 2012 John Wiley & Sons, Ltd. Published 2012 by Blackwell Publishing Ltd.

- Waste products should be disposed of following the guidelines set out in the 'Deposit of Poisonous Waste Act 1972'
- Regular cleaning and maintenance should be carried out on all processors
- Replenishment replaces used and tired chemistry each time a new film is placed into the processor
- The darkroom should be used solely for the processing of films
- The darkroom should be light-tight with reflective walls, floor and ceilings to utilise the available safelight
- Safelights are essential to prevent the fogging of films
- Handling of film under a safelight should be kept to a minimum to prevent fogging
- Safelights can be direct or indirect
- Images can be stored through thermal imaging, Polaroid images and development or the use of a video

Introduction

The processing of a radiograph is dependent on suitable equipment and its safe and efficient use. The chemistry involved is common to both manual and automatic processing, and a basic understanding of its function will assist in development of accurate and effective processing skills.

The stages of processing

The processing cycle has four main stages, regardless of whether the processing is automatic or manual. The aim of the cycle is to produce a radiograph with a diagnostic image that can be immediately viewed and stored for future reference (Figure 11.1).

The four stages are:

1 Development
2 Fixing
3 Washing
4 Drying

Development

This is the first stage. During this stage, the latent image is converted into a visible image. During development, the exposed silver halide grains are reduced to metallic silver, whilst the grains in the emulsion unaffected by the exposure do not change. This occurs through chemical reduction. The developer solution donates electrons to the

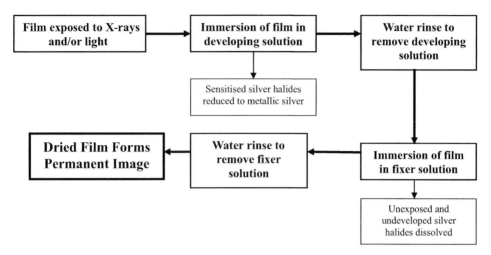

Figure 11.1   The effect of processing on the X-ray film emulsion.

silver ions in the silver halide, converting them to atoms of metallic silver. The sensitivity speck formed during exposure allows electrons from the developer to penetrate the grain and reduce the silver ions to metallic silver. If the film spends too much time in the developer solution, the developer solution may be able to penetrate unexposed grains, causing chemical fogging to the resultant film.

Fixing

This stage in processing will stop further development from occurring. This is achieved by ensuring that the solution is acidic, therefore providing a solution that will not allow the developing agents to work. Fixer will clear the image by removing silver halide crystals from the emulsion. The exposed crystals of silver halide have been converted to metallic silver but the unexposed crystals remain. Unexposed silver halide grains account for about 60% of the total number of grains in the emulsion. These crystals will still be photosensitive and will darken as time goes by. This darkening will spoil the image. During fixing, these silver halide crystals are converted to a compound that is soluble in water allowing them to dissolve out of the emulsion. The time taken for this to occur is known as the clearing time.

Clearing time	The time taken for a film to lose its milky appearance (image becomes transparent)
Fixing time	1.3 × clearing time

In the final stages, fixing will prevent any further reactions from occurring to the film emulsion and ensure that the film emulsion hardens. The fixer hardens the gelatine ensuring that it does not absorb too much water. This will in turn reduce the drying time necessary. Hardening will ensure that the emulsion is protected from damage during the washing and drying process and during the viewing and storage of the film.

Washing

Washing is essential to prevent the continuing action of the chemicals used during both developing and processing.

In manual processing, a wash tank is necessary between the developing and fixing stages. This will dilute the developer so that it will stop working and will also prevent contamination of the fixer.

During any form of processing, a final wash is necessary. If the residue substances from development and fixing are not removed, the film will gradually develop a yellow-brown (sepia) stain during storage. Dissolved salts may also crystallise on the surface of the film during storage if the film is not adequately washed.

The wash stage will only be effective if the amount of contamination in the water is lower than that in the emulsion. For this reason, it is essential that running, fresh water is used.

The efficiency of the washing process will be affected by the amount of contaminant in the emulsion, the condition of the fixer, the flow and amount of water movement, the temperature of the water and the time taken to wash the film.

In automatic processing, this time is usually about 10–20 seconds, in manual processing, a minimum of 10 minutes is essential.

If the film is left in water for too long, the emulsion may separate from the base, so careful monitoring is necessary.

Drying

During the drying process, all of the surface water and most of the water from the emulsion must be removed. The drying time will depend on a number of factors including the wetness of the emulsion and the drying conditions (humidity, temperature and air circulation). If the drying temperature is too high, the film will become brittle. In automatic processing, a squeegee will remove the surface water and evaporation will remove the water from the emulsion. This takes approximately 25 seconds. If the films are being manually dried, the films can be placed on a washing line in a dust-free environment or in a hot air cabinet. The temperature should meet the manufacturer's requirements.

Developer

Developing agents

The active agents in developer are hydroquinone and phenidone and are used in combination depending on the manufacturer's requirements. Both reduce exposed silver bromide crystals to metallic silver by the donation of electrons. No developer is completely selective, so the agents that reduce exposed crystals the quickest is used. These agents have a strong smell and can cause staining to clothing and can cause dermatitis if they are in contact for any period of time. When the two compounds are used together, the oxidation of hydroquinone will kick start the phenidone. This is known as superadditivity.

Preservative

This will slow the deterioration of the developer by producing an inert (un reactive) sulphonate that will slow the oxidation of the developer that usually occurs over time. The preservative is usually potassium metabisulphate.

Accelerator

This will maintain the alkalinity of the developer solution at about a pH of 9.6–10 (neutral is pH 7). An alkali solution will increase the rate of chemical reaction, and maintenance of the pH at these levels will give adequate speed while still controlling the activity of the developer. The compound used is usually either sodium or potassium hydroxide.

Restrainer

This will improve the selectivity of the developer, reducing the levels of chemical fogging. The development process produces potassium bromide, which is a good restrainer or a more powerful restrainer; benzotriazole can be added in the manufacture process.

Sequestering agents

These are added to the developer to prevent the build-up of a calcium sludge that may effect the processing of the film. This is usually EDTA (ethylene-diamine-tetra-acetic acid) or a sodium salt.

Solvent

The solvent in developer is water. This dissolves the developer chemicals and all the processing by-products. The water will also make the emulsion layer swell allowing the developing agents to penetrate the emulsion and reach the silver halide crystals more easily.

Other additions

Hardener reduces the emulsion swelling and softens the emulsion. A wetting agent reduces the surface tension of the developer and will also prevent frothing of the surface. A fungicide will also prevent or reduce fungal growth.

S	**Solvent**
O	**Other additives**
A	**Accelerator**
P	**Preservatives**
R	**Restrainer**
A	**A buffer**
D	**Developing agents**
S	**Sequestering agent**

Fixer

The use of a fixer will give a permanent image and stop development. The fixer solution must be able to convert unexposed silver bromide into a form that can be washed off. This is known as conversion. It must have no effect on exposed crystals.

Fixing agent

This agent will diffuse into the emulsion and will react with the silver halides. This will produce silver sulphate, ammonium bromide and ammonium argento-thiosulphate. The compound used is ammonium thiosulphate as it is cheap and easy to prepare. It will also penetrate into the film quickly reducing the chances of the film fogging. The ammonium thiosulphate will change the unexposed areas of the film from a milky white to a transparent appearance.

Solvent

The solvent used is water. This has a neutral pH and is cheap as well as readily available. This will dissolve into the emulsion carrying with it the dissolved fixer chemicals.

Acidifier

The acidifier will stop development preventing dichroic fog. This is seen as a green/blue tinged stain when the image is viewed in reflective light and a pink stain when viewed with transmitted light. The deposit of very fine silver particles causes this over the surface of the film. The acidifier will neutralise the alkali developer.

The acidifier will also allow the hardener to work. This is pH dependent and so acetic acid with a pH of 4–4.5 is used.

Buffer

This will maintain the pH of the fixer solution to within 0.2. Sodium acetate is usually used.

Preservative

This prevents decomposition of the fixer. As the ammonium thiosulphate breaks down, sulphur is formed that will stop the fixer from working. The preservative is usually sodium sulphite, which is pH dependent.

Hardener

This will prevent damage to the film and allows drying. It is composed of an aluminium salt that will prevent the emulsion from swelling excessively. It will also prevent the emulsion from softening in the wash water or during the drying process.

Anti-sludging agent

The hardener will produce insoluble compounds that will form sludge on the bottom of the tank. Boric acid is used to reduce and prevent the formation of this sludge layer.

P	Preservative
A	Acidifier
F	Fixing agent
B	Buffer
A	Anti-sludging agent
S	Solvent
H	Hardener

Parts of the automatic processor

Automatic processing works on the same principle as manual processing except that it is carried out by a machine with a series of rollers and the dry to dry time is usually much quicker than with manual processing. The automatic processor is usually simple to operate and maintain.

Film transport system

The film is initially taken into the processor through a film feed system. This will contain a microswitch that detects the film and will calculate the correct amount of replenishment required. The microswitch will also detect when the film is totally in the processor and indicate that another film can be entered or the white light can be switched back on. The film is carried through the tanks through a series of rollers. These will press the solution onto the surface of the film and will also squeegee excess chemistry off the surface of the film as it leaves the tanks (Figure 11.2). To alter the amount of time the film spends in each tank, the depth of the tank is altered, rather than having a complicated gear system. The transportation may either be vertically through a series of deep tanks or horizontally through a series of shallow trays.

Water systems and drainage

Water within the processor will assist in the control of temperature. If the water is not switched on with the processor, the developer and fixer solutions will overheat and will not work effectively. The temperature used in automatic processors is usually higher than that for manual processing. The water for washing is usually cold although slightly warm water is more efficient. To prevent the formation of algae, the water is on timer control so that it is constantly changed and moved through the system.

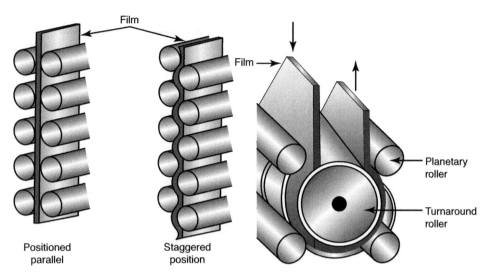

Figure 11.2 Roller system from a processor.

The drainage of water and other products from the processor are controlled by the 'Deposit of Poisonous Waste Act 1972' and these must be adhered to carefully. The developer and fixer solutions should not enter the public sewer without the consent of the local authority and, if possible, the waste fixer and developer should be stored and disposed of separately through a recognised company who deal in waste chemicals.

Dryer systems

The film is dried using hot air at 50–60°C. The air is warmed either by an electric heater or infrared lamps surrounded by air blowers. On entry into the dryer, more rollers squeegee the film so the water to be removed from the film is minimal (Figure 11.3).

Care of the automatic processor

The automatic processor needs as much care and cleaning as a manual processor if not more. The tanks and rollers must be cleaned regularly (once a week) to stop build-up of the residual chemicals that may impair the function of the processor. The build-up of residual chemicals will speed up the deterioration of the remaining chemicals, may cause scratches to the film and may cause the film to override the rollers. Details of cleaning and maintenance regimes are usually supplied with the processor.

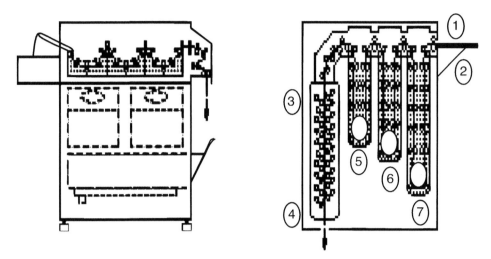

Figure 11.3   Horizontal and vertical automatic processors.

Replenishment

Replenishment is an essential part of the maintenance of the processor whether it is manual or automatic. General radiography will result in about 40% of the silver on the film being used. The remainder will be washed out into the developer and fixer solution along with the by-products of the processing cycle, leading to a reduction in the concentration of the developer and fixer. The amount of replenishment will depend on the throughput of X-rays. As throughput increases, the amount of replenishment for each film will decrease, as there is less time for the solutions to degenerate. If a thicker emulsion is used, then more chemicals will be carried over from one tank to another and the amount of replenishment for each film will need to be increased.

Replenishment during manual processing

Replenishment is not easy with manual processing and the levels of chemistry in the respective tanks should be monitored and topped up. The average life of developer is about 10 weeks, regardless of the amount of use. Even without any use, the condition of the developer will deteriorate.

If the throughput is low, it may be more economical to dish develop films and only make up 1-gallon containers of fixer and developer. This can then be decanted into litter trays or other similar containers when required. The fixer and developer can then be discarded after use. The pre-made containers of fixer and developer can be stored at room temperature out of direct sunlight until they are needed.

Replenishment in an automatic processor

Every time a film is fed into the processor, the entry roller system will trigger the replenishment system. This will allow replenisher solution to be pumped into the tanks in the processor. The new solution is mixed with the old by the action of the rollers and excess drains out through an overflow into the silver recovery unit and the drainage system. The replenishment chemicals are held in reservoir tanks or in smaller units in plastic containers. Maximum efficiency can be obtained through the use of an automixer. This is a unit that will automatically mix the fresh chemistry and store it until it is required by the processor. This is much cleaner and saves time when compared to manual mixing. It will also ensure accurate and total mixing of the chemicals and water.

Starter solution and mixing chemicals

When the processor is started from dry, a starter solution containing potassium bromide and acetic acid is needed. This will depress the pH of the developer, decreasing the activity of the solution. This will control the activity of the developing agents and increase the selectivity of the new developer solution.

Developer is usually supplied in two or three containers containing the main constituents that are mixed with water.

Fixer comes in two separate containers: Part A contains the replenisher with most of the chemicals and Part B contains the hardener. This hardener can cause burns and allergies if it is inhaled. If Parts A and B are stored together, they will deteriorate and should only be put in the same container when they are required for use.

Silver recovery

Silver can be recovered from either used fixer solution or from old, discarded films. The films and fixer solution can be collected and recycled by a firm that specialises in refining silver. If the radiographic throughput of the veterinary practice is constant, the cost of removing the films and used fixer solution will be compensated by the amount of silver recovered. Once the silver recovery has taken place, depending on the methods used, the fixer solution can be reused. Approximately 98% of the total silver in fixer solution can be reclaimed. This can be carried out using electrolysis or the depositing of silver on a steel wool column.

As the sources of silver become scarcer, recovery of used silver in this form is essential to reduce the cost of industrial silver and maintain silver for future generations.

The darkroom

The darkroom is the room where films are processed or placed into the automatic processor and the area in which cassettes will be reloaded. It will also provide a safe area for the handling of films. The room should be easily accessible to all. It should not be near any damp or hot areas with good ventilation and must have a reliable source of electricity and water. The room must be away from any sources of direct or scattered radiation.

If manual processing is taking place, the darkroom should have distinct wet and dry areas so that contamination of films and screens does not take place. The dry area (present in both manual and automatic processing environments) should have a workbench where cassettes can be opened and closed easily. The bench should be made of wood or linoleum so that static build-up is avoided. Film storage should be available in the dry area either in the form of a hopper or light tight drawers. Boxes of films should not be stored on the work surfaces.

The wet area should contain the manual processor or tanks and the drying area. This should be separate from the dry area (Figure 11.4).

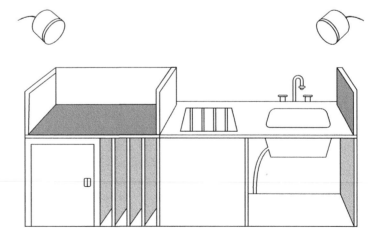

Figure 11.4   Layout of a darkroom with dry and wet areas.

Size

The room should have a minimum floor space of 10 m^2. This will provide adequate room to move around and safely use the manual processing tanks and film hoppers or drawers storing the films.

Floors

The floor should be light-coloured, composed of a non-porous, non-slip material that can be easily cleaned and maintained. As the environment is usually poorly lit, trip hazards should not be present and obstacles should be kept to a minimum.

Walls and ceilings

The walls should be light to reflect as much safelight as possible into the room and onto the working surfaces. This may reduce the number of light fittings required to give a suitable intensity of light to work with. The walls should be easy to keep clean and in wet processing areas they should be tiled for easy maintenance and cleaning.

Ceilings should be white or cream and a paint that could flake (emulsion) should be avoided.

Ventilation

The room should be well ventilated to provide a safe and comfortable environment for staff. The area should not be too hot or humid as this could damage the films stored in the room.

Doors

Where a single door is used, care must be taken to ensure accidental entry during processing is avoided. The door should be light-sealed and have a lock or some description. If there is space, a double-door system is ideal. This involves two doors that will provide a light lock. The walls should be painted black to prevent the reflection of light into the dark room. If the room has windows, there should be black light proof blinds provided that run in channels to prevent the light penetrating round the edges of the blinds.

White lights

White lights are needed in the darkroom to allow safe and thorough cleaning of the floor and work surfaces. The white light is also needed for the safe maintenance and cleaning of the processor and any other equipment needed in the dark room. The lights should not be fluorescent as these give an afterglow that could cause fogging. Two switches should be provided. A light switch is needed near the door with a second switch nearer to the work surfaces. The switches should be away from the safelight switches or marked in some easily distinguishable way.

Safelights

A safelight is essential to prevent light affecting the film and causing fogging. All radiographic film is sensitive to white light and so the light must be filtered. A safelight is a box containing a low wattage (maximum of 25-W pearl light bulb) and a filter to remove the parts of the spectrum that the film is most sensitive to. The filter is a layer of gelatine, dyed to the appropriate colour between two sheets of glass. Most radiographic film is sensitive to green or blue light and so selecting a filter that will remove this light will result in reduced fogging of the film (Figure 11.5).

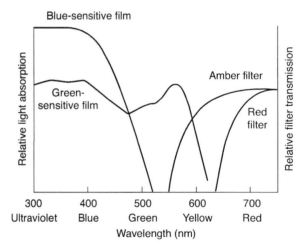

Figure 11.5   The effect of safelight colour on light transmission.

Even with the use of suitable safelights, fogging of the film will occur and the efficiency of the safelights should be monitored. If a safelight becomes cracked, it will cause fogging to the radiographs. Handling of films under safelight conditions should be kept to a minimum, as fogging and a loss of contrast will eventually be seen on all films.

Direct safelights

This is usually in the form of a beehive safelight. This will direct the light straight onto the work surface and the film. This type of safelight should be at least 1.2 m from the work surface. This type of safelight is the most suitable type of light for area in which cassettes are loaded and unloaded (Figure 11.6).

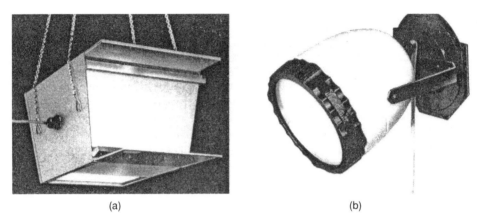

(a)   (b)

Figure 11.6   (a) Indirect (hanging) safelight; (b) direct (beehive) safelight.

Indirect safelighting

This type of safelight will give general illumination to the darkroom. The light is directed towards the ceiling and is then reflected back into the room. The safelight will usually have filters above and below providing direct and indirect illumination. These should be at least 2.1 m above the floor of the darkroom (Figure 11.6).

Control of substances hazardous to health (COSHH) regulations

The chemicals involved in the developing of X-ray films are hazardous if inhaled or splashed on the skin. Great care should be taken when replenishing the tanks and during cleaning. Masks and gloves should always be worn and there should be adequate ventilation at all times in the room surrounding the processor. Allergies can develop over time if there is unregulated exposure to the fumes given off by the chemicals.

Other methods of processing

The effect of X-rays can be demonstrated on media other than conventional radiographic film. This is a good solution if processing facilities are not available especially during theatre cases using fluoroscopy or when working in remote locations away from conventional processing facilities.

Polaroid

Polaroid imaging uses a special type of film that works in reverse to conventional radiographic film. The Polaroid film usually comes in a pack with negative and positive films and a pod of jellified processing chemicals. The film is exposed in the usual way and then placed into a custom-made processor. This will use a series of rollers to break the pod of chemicals and spread it evenly over the film. The latent image is formed in the silver halide of the negative sheet. During processing, the jellified chemicals will develop both exposed and unexposed silver halides in the negative emulsion. Areas on the negative that have received an exposure will have black silver deposited; the unexposed areas will donate silver ions to the crystalline silver layer on the positive film. This is the image that will be viewed. It will be the reverse to the negative image.

Thermal imaging

The image is produced by heat. Light produces a latent image on special heat sensitive paper and then it is developed using heat. This dries the silver in the paper to form the image. Thermal imaging can be used to print a radiographic image from a television monitor. This is of use during fluoroscopic examinations where no other means of image storage or retrieval (10 cm film or video) is available.

Video

Video images can be used to store a real-time image (as it happens) during fluoroscopy. This gives the option to view the procedure repeatedly and actually requires a lower patient dose. The main disadvantage of this method is a reduction in image resolution.

Further reading

Easton, S. (2002) The ideal darkroom. *Veterinary Nursing* 17(6), 213–216.
This article expands the discussion on the darkroom and the use of safelights.

Revision questions

1 Give in order the four main stages of processing.

2 Describe what happens to the exposed silver halide crystals during development.

3 What factors will affect the efficiency of the washing process?

4 Name the two compounds in developing solution.

5 Why is water used as the solvent in fixer solution?

6 How does the film transport system of an automatic processor work?

7 Give two uses for water in an automatic processor.

8 Describe the daily care needed to maintain an automatic processor.

9 How does replenishment in an automatic processor work?

10 How does a safelight work?

Chapter 12

Digital Radiography

Chapter contents

Computed radiography
Care of the imaging plate and cassette
Computerised radiography process
Digital radiography
Image storage
Image display
Image quality
Further reading

Key points

- Digital imaging is slowly replacing film radiography
- Digital radiography uses an image receptor that produces the image without the need for a reader
- Computerised radiography uses an image receiver that is placed in a reader to allow viewing of the image
- Images can be viewed rapidly
- Manipulation of images is possible
- Images can be stored in digital format, reducing storage requirements within the practice

Introduction

Digital imaging has already been in use for many years in computed tomography (CT), magnetic resonance imaging (MRI), nuclear medicine (NM), fluoroscopy and ultrasound, but only recently conventional X-ray equipment has started using digital technology. Many veterinary practices are replacing conventional processors and cassettes with computerised radiography (Figure 12.1).

The main advantage is that images can be viewed rapidly, manipulated quickly and then sent to a computer network for reporting and

Practical Veterinary Diagnostic Imaging, Second Edition. Suzanne Easton.
© 2012 John Wiley & Sons, Ltd. Published 2012 by Blackwell Publishing Ltd.

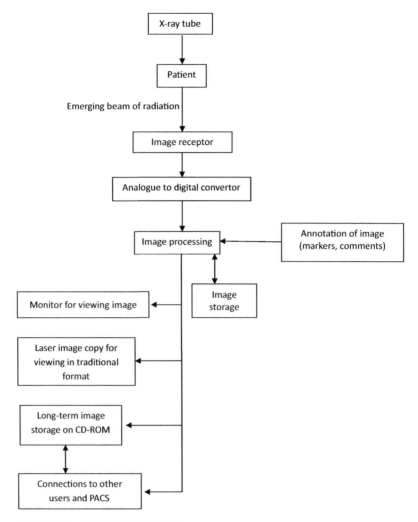

Figure 12.1   Digital imaging chart.

viewing. Storage space is greatly reduced due to the absence of films, and images can be sent to specialists and clients easily.

Digital radiography has greater exposure latitude than X-ray film. Over- and underexposure will still be visible on the resultant image. However, there is a trade-off between radiation dose and image quality. High exposures give a very clear image but with an unacceptable dose to the patient. Low exposures result in a noisy (grainy) image and may result in important information being missed (Figure 12.2).

There are two types of digital imaging currently in use: computed radiography (CR) and digital radiography (DR).

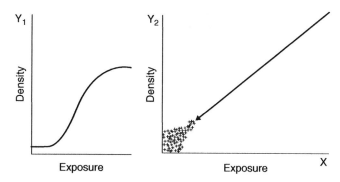

Figure 12.2   A characteristic curve for conventional film, compared to that of digital imaging.

Computed radiography

Computed radiography provides a direct replacement for practices that have been using conventional film, without the need to replace the X-ray tube and related equipment. It uses storage phosphor cassettes, which directly replaces a conventional cassette with film and intensifying screen.

The imaging plate

The imaging plate is the replacement in computerised radiography for the conventional cassette. The imaging plate is coated with photostimulable phosphors (PSPs) that capture X-rays after exposure of the patient (Figure 12.3).

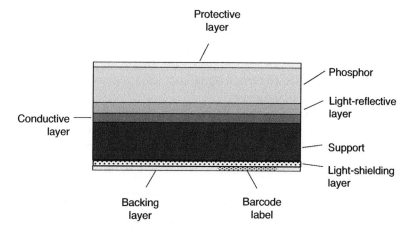

Figure 12.3   Construction of the imaging plate.

The PSP material stores the irradiated energy and then releases the energy as visible light in response to the stimulation of a beam of laser light. Europium-doped barium fluorohalides are used. These are either chlorine-, bromine- or iodine-based.

As the X-rays pass through the PSP material, they interact with the electrons in the fluorohalide crystals, giving them energy. This enables the electrons to enter the conduction band. Some electrons return to the valence band, but others remain between the two bands. This trapped signal is proportional to the amount of radiation that the plate has received, and it is these electrons that form the latent image (Figure 12.4).

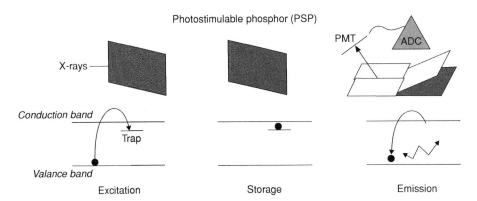

Figure 12.4 Schematic sequence of images of conduction and valence bands showing 'trapped' electrons.

Retrieving the latent image

A CR reader is used to extract the latent image from the plate. A laser scans the plate, giving the electrons enough energy to return to the correct position. This process results in blue light being emitted. This light is collected and passes through a photomultiplier tube where it is amplified to form a signal that can be viewed on a monitor and stored in a digital format.

The light moves through the photomultiplier, is then amplified and then the signal is digitised using an analogue-to-digital converter, allowing temporary storage of the image in digital format. This can then be sent to a monitor for viewing or to a printer (Figure 12.5).

Erasure of the plate

After the image has been retrieved, some electrons remain trapped. These remaining electrons are removed using a bright white light.

This is done after each image has been retrieved and should also be carried out periodically to prevent a build-up of background signals.

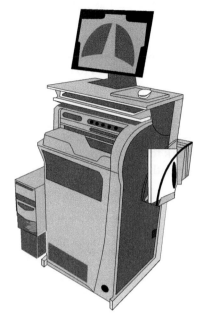

Figure 12.5   Schematic diagram of a CR plate reader.

Care of the imaging plate and cassette

Cleaning and maintenance procedures should be followed to ensure that the warranty on the imaging plate is not invalidated. Following these procedures will also extend the life of the image receiver and plate.

Computed radiography plates should be regularly checked as part of a quality assurance programme for damage. The imaging plates also need regular checks, as the edges get damaged and cracks can appear, and they can be vulnerable to scratches. The cassette catches should also be checked to ensure the plate does not drop out whilst being used.

Computerised radiography process

All systems work in a slightly different manner, and time should be taken to raise your awareness of the systems in place. The plate is linked to the patient using the barcode and a unique identification is used for the patient. X-rays are taken in the conventional manner using a normal X-ray machine, and the film cassette is replaced with a CR plate. The operator then identifies the examinations completed on the CR reader, and the plates are placed into the reader. The examination selection is important as it will ensure the correct protocol is used for image processing. The reader will identify the patient from the barcode and allocate the images to the patient.

The CR reader removes the plate from the cassette and this is read, erased and then returned to the operator. The image is then viewed on an acquisition workstation, cropped and markers applied. The image can be checked for quality and dose indicators such as sensitivity or exposure index. Once the operator is satisfied that the image is correctly identified, manipulated and annotated, it is then sent on to the network for reporting and storage for retrieval at a later date from anywhere within that network (Figure 12.6).

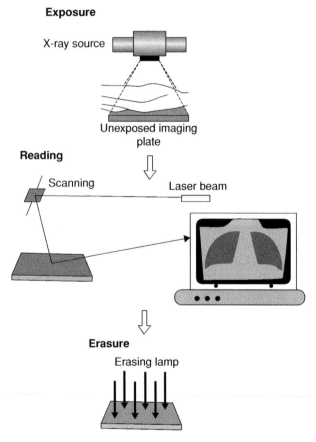

Figure 12.6 The sequence of events during a diagnostic examination using computerised radiography.

Digital radiography

There are two systems in place for DR, both of which have the image receptor as an integral part of the equipment:

1 Indirect DR (IDR) produces an analogue signal, which is converted by an analogue-to-digital converter.
2 Direct DR where the incoming X-ray photons are transformed directly into an electronic signal.

Indirect digital radiography

Indirect DR uses a phosphor called caesium iodide (CsI) that is coated over an active matrix array (AMA) of amorphous silicon (a-Si; Figure 12.7).

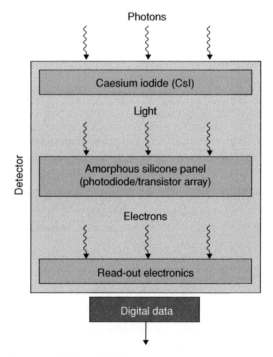

Figure 12.7   Amorphous silicon detector.

X-ray photons are absorbed by CsI and are converted into light photons. The amorphous silicon array converts the light into an electrical signal and this signal is sent to an image processor. This allows the display and storage of the image. The strength of the signal is directly proportional to the number of X-ray photon interactions that have occurred.

Disadvantages of indirect digital radiography

- *Scatter*: The amount can depend on the thickness and structure of the phosphor material; however, it will be less than screen film.
- *Noise on the image*: This can be reduced by cooling the detector.
- Systems are currently restricted by size – each image processor represents 1 pixel on the image, and images are of several megapixels or even gigapixels in size.
- Spatial resolution is restricted because of the physical size of the image processor and the pixel.

Direct digital radiography

Direct DR does not use a phosphor material. X-ray photons strike an amorphous selenium (a-Se) detector and are directly converted into an electrical charge. The amorphous selenium is coated on a thin-film-transistor (TFT) array (Figure 12.8). As the X-rays pass through, they generate positive and negative charges between the detectors, which are in proportion to the level of X-ray exposure. The positive charges are drawn to the capacitor where they are stored and read out by the electronics within the array.

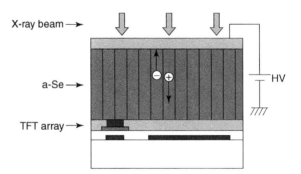

Figure 12.8   Amorphous selenium detector.

Advantages of direct digital radiography

- Better spatial resolution compared to IDR, as there is no scatter in the phosphor layer.
- Greater efficiency, as there is only one energy conversion as compared to the two needed for IDR.
- Simpler design, so manufacturing is easier.
- No need for a separate photodetector for each pixel.

Disadvantages of direct digital radiography

- Detector is very temperature-dependent, and extremes of heat or cold can cause damage to it.

- Detector is fragile and is not suited to all aspects of veterinary work.
- The imaging plate is made up from lots of detectors, so there sometimes can be differences between them. Software can be used to smooth out the differences. This is called 'stitching'.

Image storage

Every DR system will have a slightly different method of recording and storing images. The most common method is PACS (picture archiving and communications system). This can be used for image acquisition, image display, the network, storage and retrieval of images in most clinical environments (Figure 12.9).

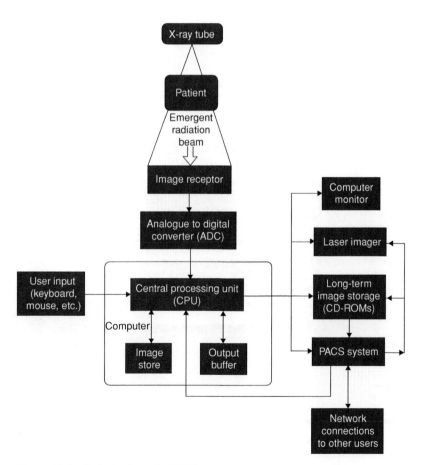

Figure 12.9   Typical set-up of a PACS.

Image display

The initial reporting display system must be able to manage large data files and demonstrate the images at full resolution and with all greyscale levels visible. There should be a fast response to manipulation of the images. For subsequent image reviewing, the high quality is not so important, so standard PC monitors are acceptable.

The image display should be part of a quality assurance programme to ensure viewing conditions remain satisfactory throughout the monitor's lifespan. The reporting monitors must be checked daily using a recognised test pattern such as the SMPTE test pattern (Figure 12.10).

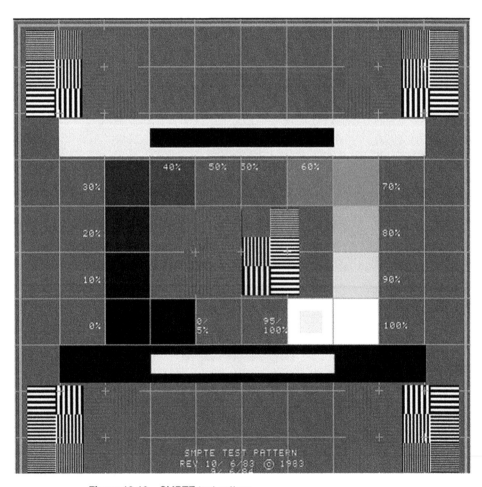

Figure 12.10   SMPTE test pattern.

Image quality

Digital radiography produces far fewer faults; however, they can still occur. They fall into three main categories: hardware, software and object.

Hardware artefacts

Hardware faults occur due to an error in the process involved in the use of the plate, reader or the hard-copy printer. Most are transient and are due to the non-erased (phantom) images, dust or dirt and can be rectified with cleaning and full erasure of the plate.

Skipped scan lines or distorted images can occur if there is a malfunction with the image reader, and over time the laser will lose power and will need to be replaced.

Software artefacts

Care should be taken to select the correct processing option. Incorrect selection will result in the wrong algorithm being applied, resulting in non-diagnostic images. The algorithms may cause problems in some units if more than one image is exposed on a plate.

Object artefacts

These artefacts usually arise because of the following:

- Object mispositioning.
- Scan line interference patterns with the grid, which results in moiré patterns.
- A 'halo' effect that can appear around the edges of objects and is caused by the unsharp masking technique if performed incorrectly.
- Backscatter that can contribute significantly to contrast degradation.

Further reading

Oakley, J. (2003) *Digital Imaging*. Cambridge: Cambridge University Press.
This textbook provides a detailed review of digital imaging.

Revision questions

1 What does PSP stand for?

2 How is the PSP plate read once it has been exposed to X-rays?

3 What are the differences between indirect digital radiography and computerised radiography?

4 What is PACS and how can it be used in veterinary practice?

5 Identify two faults that can occur in digital imaging.

Chapter 13

Radiographic Image Quality

Chapter contents

Sensitometry
Densitometry
Characteristic curve
Latitude
Density
Contrast
Magnification
Distortion
Movement
Producing a high-quality radiograph
Commonly seen film faults
Further reading

Key points

- Sensitometry assesses the performance of films, film–screen combinations or a processor
- Sensitometry results are recorded to form a characteristic curve
- Latitude is the range of exposures that will ensure a diagnostic image on a radiographic film
- Density is the degree of blackening on a film
- Contrast is the difference in density between two adjacent structures
- Magnification occurs if the distance between the object and the film is large
- Distortion occurs if the object being imaged is not parallel to the primary beam
- Movement can cause blurring and reduction in sharpness of the film
- Film faults have a detrimental effect on image quality and can be eliminated by care and maintenance of equipment

Practical Veterinary Diagnostic Imaging, Second Edition. Suzanne Easton.
© 2012 John Wiley & Sons, Ltd. Published 2012 by Blackwell Publishing Ltd.

Introduction

During the production of radiographs, a number of faults can occur, which can be categorised as either human or mechanically generated. These can be detrimental to the diagnostic value of the radiograph. Through simple quality assurance and equipment care, these faults can be avoided and, if they do occur, identified at an early stage to prevent unnecessary repeat radiographs and possible extended anaesthesia for the patient.

Sensitometry

Sensitometry is a way of assessing the performance of a film, screen, film–screen combination or a processor. To allow successful sensitometry, a sensitometry strip needs to be produced by using a sensitometer. The sensitometer is a device containing a controlled light source and filters. The combination of the light and filters simulates the effect of light from the intensifying screens on a film. A step wedge can be used to provide a scale of graduated densities for sensitometry. The step wedge is a strip of aluminium with varying thickness of additional metal. Both the step wedge and sensitometer produce an image with varying shades of grey. The exposure should always be made using the same machine or exposure factors. If these factors alter, then the density of the steps may alter, possibly leading to inaccurate analysis.

Densitometry

The density of the film is assessed using a densitometer. The densitometer compares the intensity of light incident on and transmitted through a selected area of film. This is known as the optical density. The details received through the use of the densitometer can be recorded and plotted. This gives a characteristic curve.

Sensitometry	**Means of assessing film, screen or processor function**
Sensitometer	**A device used to produce a range of densities ready for analysis**
Step wedge	**Aluminium strips of increasing thickness Exposed to produce a range of densities for analysis**
Densitometer	**Device used to assess the incident light falling on and transmitted through a radiographic film**

Characteristic curve

The results obtained from the densitometer can be plotted to produce a characteristic curve. The curve is plotted on a graph to show the relative exposure against the density. Using a mathematical calculation involving the log of the relative exposure compresses the scale to give a suitable graph and ensures that two exposures always have the same separation on the exposure scale. The relative exposure is obtained from the exposures used in the production of the step wedge. From the graph, the useful density of the film, the film latitude and exposure latitude can be calculated.

When the data are plotted, the graph has three distinct areas: the shoulder, toe and straight-line portion (Figure 13.1). At the toe and shoulder, large variations in exposure factors result in very small changes in the optical density.

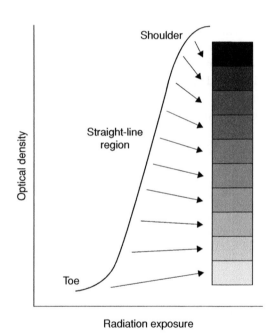

Figure 13.1   Characteristic curve of radiographic film.

Toe

At the toe, the levels of optical density are just above the base density and fog. In this region, very small changes in density will result from changes in exposure factors. The toe is the area of underexposure on a diagnostic radiograph.

Straight-line portion

In the straight-line portion, the image will be properly exposed and can be used to form a diagnostic image.

Shoulder

The shoulder is the area of the curve where further increases in exposure produce gradually smaller increases in density. This is the region of overexposure.

Latitude

The latitude of a film describes the range of exposures that will ensure that a diagnostic image is possible. This can be determined from the characteristic curve, but is determined by the manufacturer. If a film has wide latitude, there is a greater range of exposure factors that will produce a diagnostic image. If the film has narrow latitude, then the response of the film is more limited. Films with wide latitude will have longer grey scales than films with narrow latitude. If the film has a high contrast, it will have narrow latitude (less grey range; Figure 13.2).

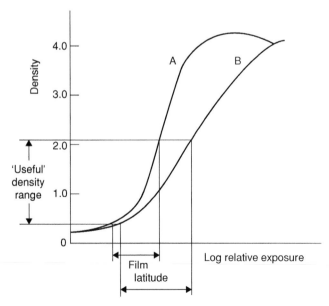

Figure 13.2   Characteristic curves for high- and low-latitude film–screen imaging system.

Density

The density of a film describes the amount of blackening on the resultant image. This subject density is related to the density of the part being examined (Figure 13.3).

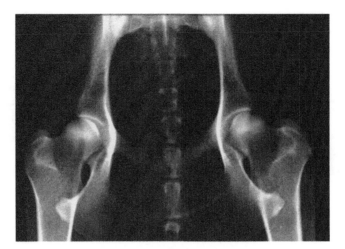

Figure 13.3   A radiograph of the pelvis showing a range of densities.

If a part of the patient is very dense and has a high atomic number, for example bone, the number of X-ray photons passing through it will be low. This will result in a pale or clear area on the radiograph. If the area of interest is not dense, such as the lung, and has a low atomic number, such as that of air, the X-rays will pass through easily and will cause areas of blackness on the film (Table 13.1).

Table 13.1   Radiographic density and appearance of different tissues.

Tissue	Density	Atomic number	Appearance on X-ray
Bone	High	High	White
Water/muscle	Medium/high	High	Grey
Fat	Low/medium	Low	Grey
Air	Low	Low	Black

Photographic density may also be present because of fogging on the radiographic film due to storage conditions, processing conditions or light exposure.

Contrast

The term contrast describes the density between two adjacent structures on a radiographic image. If there is a wide range of grey on the image but very little black and white, the image has a long scale of contrast. If there are a lot of black and white areas but limited greys on a radiographic image, then the image has a short scale of contrast (Figure 13.4).

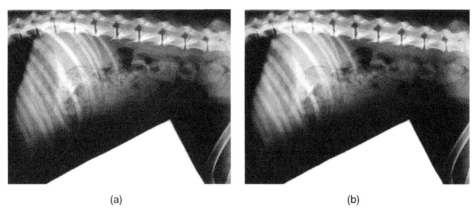

(a)   (b)

Figure 13.4   (a) High- and (b) low-contrast images showing range of grey tones.

In diagnostic radiography, a long contrast scale is ideal, giving a wide range of grey but limited black and white on the image. Films that have a short scale of contrast will have a narrow range of latitude.

The contrast of a film is dependent on a number of factors:

- Tissue density and atomic number
- Kilovoltage
- Object shape and thickness
- Film contrast
- Film fogging
- Use of contrast medium

All of these factors will alter the contrast of the image, although the degree each part plays is difficult to define.

Tissue density and atomic number

These two factors are closely related. An increase in atomic number and density will result in more X-ray photons being absorbed. If the tissue being radiographed is dense, then a higher kV_p will be required. This will result in higher X-ray energy and the presence of Compton scatter and the photoelectric effect. If the tissue has a lower density, such as soft tissue and fat, then the kV_p required to penetrate the tissue will be lower.

Kilovoltage

This is the most variable exposure factor when contrast is being determined. As the kV_p increases, the contrast scale increases. The use of a high kV_p will produce a wide range of grey scale (long scale of contrast). A low kV_p will produce an image with a lot of blacks and whites but a limited grey scale. The use of a low kV_p will need the use of higher mAs to produce an image of a similar density. This is not desirable, as it will increase the patient dose. An increased kV is used in chest radiography to 'flatten' the image and improve the contrast. In most situations, the kV should be increased rather than time, as movement blur with longer exposure times will reduce the image contrast.

Object shape and thickness

The shape and thickness of the body will alter the contrast of the radiographic image. If the area is very thin, it will absorb less X-rays than an area with greater thickness. This can lead to uneven contrast across a radiograph and even through an organ if the thickness alters. This is seen in abdominal radiographs of deep-chested and thin dogs. The contrast is acceptable in one region (cranial or caudal), but the second area appears to be lacking in contrast due to a different thickness or absence of tissue. This can be overcome by placing lead shielding in the area of the primary beam in the caudal abdomen to fill in the area of missing tissue. This will increase the contrast of the caudal abdomen. The problem can also be overcome by taking two separate radiographs with different exposure factors to demonstrate the two areas.

Film contrast

The film contrast describes the latitude of a film. Films with a wide range of latitude will have a higher contrast giving a wider range of grey scale. This is due to the silver halide crystal shape or size in the film emulsion.

Film fogging

Film fogging is caused by poor storage of films or exposure to light or radiation including scattered radiation during the examination. Fogging causes the film to have an overall greyness and a reduction in contrast.

Use of contrast medium

The contrast of an image can be improved through the use of contrast medium. All contrast media have high atomic numbers (iodine = 53, barium = 56) and these will absorb more X-ray photons. If the exposure factors are not altered to accommodate this absorption, then the contrast of the radiographic image will be enhanced. If a negative contrast medium (air) is introduced, then exposure factors will need to be reduced to maintain the contrast on the radiographic image.

Contrast on a radiograph can be altered by:

- **Tissue density and atomic number**
- **Kilovoltage**
- **Object shape and thickness**
- **Film contrast**
- **Film fogging**
- **Use of contrast medium**

Magnification

If the distance between the object being radiographed and the film is very large, magnification will occur. This is due to the primary beam continuing to diverge once it has passed through the object. This distorts the image and makes it appear larger than it actually is. This can be used to our advantage in controlled situations where very small objects are being imaged using magnification. This is known as macro-radiography. The amount of magnification present can be calculated with a simple equation:

$$\text{Magnification} = \frac{\text{Focal film distance (FFD)}}{\text{Film–object distance (FOD)}}$$

If it is essential to know how much magnification has occurred, such as fracture planning a marker can be used. This marker will have a known length and can be imaged on the same film, next to the object. The magnification factor from this known size can then be applied to the object (Figure 13.5).

Distortion

Distortion occurs if the object being imaged is not parallel to the primary beam. Distortion means that the object appears elongated or foreshortened. This can be detrimental to the image quality as size

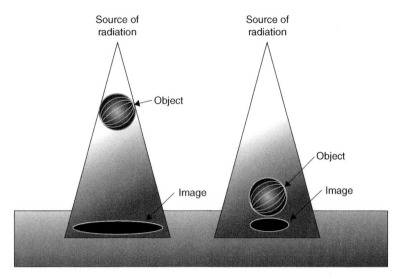

Figure 13.5 Changes in resultant image size with an increase in object–film distance.

and shape of the object cannot be calculated accurately. This will also be seen at the periphery of the image and care must be taken in interpretation of these areas (Figure 13.6).

Distortion can be used to the radiographer's advantage in preventing superimposition of structures that may otherwise be on top of each other. This is especially the case in skull examination.

Movement

Movement can have a detrimental effect on the image quality. It will result in the radiographic image being blurred, with a reduction in overall contrast and possibly magnification if the movement has been away from the film. Movement of the patient can be reduced by using the shortest possible exposure time (with a high mA), ensuring that the tube support is stable and by using restraint. Restraint can be in the form of sedation or through the use of sandbags and ties.

Image quality can be affected by:

- **Density of the image**
- **Contrast of the radiographic image**
- **Penumbra**
- **Focal spot size**
- **Anode-heel effect**
- **Magnification**
- **Distortion**
- **Movement**

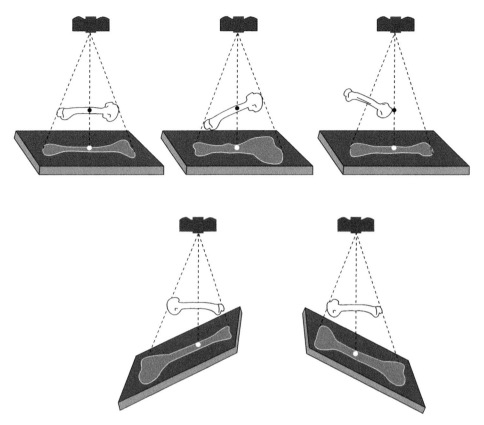

Figure 13.6   Effects of distortion on the length (or shape) of an object.

Producing a high-quality radiograph

The production of a quality radiograph must take into account all of the factors described above. A satisfactory radiograph is said to be diagnostic.

A high-quality radiograph will provide sufficient views to make a diagnosis, with adequate exposure factors and high-quality processing with no artefacts. The use of standard projections and accurate positioning with good collimation will assist in the production of a diagnostic radiograph.

To improve the quality of the radiographic image further, the animal must be free from any possible causes of artefacts. This includes dried mud, a wet coat or even spilt contrast medium if this has been administered to the animal previously. Collars, leads and dressings can also cause artefacts on the film and should be removed or moved away from the primary beam.

Commonly seen film faults

This description of film faults is not exhaustive, but provides an outline of the more common film faults seen in veterinary radiography and solutions to help improve the image quality. Technique is the most common cause of film faults and this can be due to a number of very different reasons:

- Inadequate number of projections
- Lack of collimation
- No anatomical markers
- No patient identification or date
- Poor positioning or centring
- Movement
- Incorrect use of a grid
- Poor film–screen contact
- Magnification
- Distortion
- Film/screen graininess

Appearance of film	Film fault	Reason for fault	Solution
Whole film too dark	Film overexposed	Incorrect settings	Decrease kV, mA or time
		Wrong focal film distance	Increase focal film distance
		Wrong film–screen combination	Use slower film–screen combination
Overall greyness to film	Film fogging	Film beyond expiry date	
		Poor film storage	Ensure correct storage conditions are maintained
		Film affected by scattered radiation	Ensure a grid is used, and store cassettes away from radiation

(*Continued*)

Appearance of film	Film fault	Reason for fault	Solution
		Film exposed to light	Check for stray leaks in the darkroom and ensure that the safelight is correct
	Overdevelopment	Incorrect formula	Ensure chemistry is correctly diluted
		Developer overheated	Maintain correct temperature
		Film left in developer for too long	Check immersion times carefully
		Developer contaminated with fixer	Make a fresh solution
Whole film too light	Film underexposed	Incorrect settings	Increase kV, mA or time
		Wrong focal film distance	Decrease focal film distance
		Wrong film–screen combination	Use faster film–screen combination
		Normal exposure used with a grid	
		Cassette used back to front	
Overall lightness to film	Underdevelopment	Developing time too short	Adjust developing time

(Continued)

Appearance of film	Film fault	Reason for fault	Solution
		Developer below temperature	Maintain correct temperature
		Developer too dilute	Check mixing and dilution
		Developer exhausted	Make a fresh solution
Whole film clear	No exposure	Exposure not made correctly	
		Film placed in fixer before developer	
White areas	Bright white specks or object	Material between screen and film	Clean screens
	White area as a bright spot	Chemical spill on screen	Ensure cassettes are stored closed
	White splash marks on film	Fixer splashes on film before developing	Ensure strict darkroom practice
	Fingerprint	Fingers contaminated with fixer	Make sure that hands are clean and dry before handling films
	White area (not bright)	Contrast medium on coat or table	After contrast examinations or spillage, ensure thorough cleaning is carried out
	Straight clear strip at top of film	Developer tank levels are low	Check tank levels before processing

(Continued)

Appearance of film	Film fault	Reason for fault	Solution
	Clear strip across middle of film	Scratches to emulsion of film through handling or poor processing	Handle films carefully and carry out regular cleaning of the processor
Black areas	Straight scratches or marks	Film dropped on floor or handled roughly during processing	
	Crescent marks on film	Pressure marks from fingernails	Handle film carefully
	Dots or tree pattern on film	Static electricity	Do not wear nylon Handle films carefully
	Splashes and streaks	Film splashed before processing with any liquid apart from fixer	Carefully maintain darkroom procedures
	Black, irregular border on all sides of the film	Light leakage from the edges of the cassette	Make sure cassettes are properly shut and are not damaged

(Continued)

Appearance of film	Film fault	Reason for fault	Solution
	Black strip on end of film	Light leakage	Check film storage Do not lift lid off developer tanks during processing Allow film to enter automatic processor before using white light
	Linear black lines along full length of film	Pressure from rollers in processor	Keep rollers clean Check springs on roller assembly Do not pull films out of the dryer
Manual processing problems	Streaks and runs on films	Film hangers dirty	Routinely clean hangers to prevent the build-up of chemicals
	Film dark at top with the lower half lighter	Uneven development	Always stir the developer before use
		Insufficient agitation	Move the films slightly once they are in the developer
	Film cloudy and streaky, possibly with a sticky surface	Insufficient fixing	Make sure the film has sufficient time in the fixer Change chemicals regularly

(Continued)

Appearance of film	Film fault	Reason for fault	Solution
	Brown staining all over the film	Insufficient fixing	Make sure fixing time is adequate Change fixer regularly
	Uneven yellow or pale brown staining	Insufficient washing	Wash films for at least 30 min with fresh, running water
	Grey speckles all over the exposed part of the film	Wash water stagnant and dirty	Keep tanks empty when not in use and clean regularly to prevent the build-up of algae

Further reading

Whilst there are no specific texts recommended for this area of study, time should be taken to review faults found in practice. You should be able to identify the fault through the use of the table and comments provided in this chapter.

Revision questions

1 What is the use of sensitometry and densitometry?

2 What is latitude?

3 How will bone, air, fat and water appear on a radiograph?

4 What does contrast describe?

5 If a film has a long scale of contrast, does it have wide latitude or narrow latitude?

6 An increase in what factor will cause magnification?

7 What will distortion do to a radiographic image?

8 How can movement be avoided?

9 How can an overdeveloped film be corrected on the repeat processing?

10 What type of film fault will produce bright white specks on the radiograph?

Chapter 14

Radiation Protection

Chapter contents

The effects of ionising radiation on the body
The basics to remember
Ionising Radiation Regulations 1999
Radiation safety in the veterinary practice
Classifying the areas around an X-ray machine
Dose limits
Monitoring devices
Lead shielding
Quality assurance
Further reading

Key points

- Ionising radiation damages cells
- Ionising radiation is not selective of cell type
- Immature or rapidly dividing cells are at more risk of damage
- Dose limits should not be exceeded
- Exposure to personnel should be kept to a minimum
- Unnecessary procedures should not be performed
- The Ionising Radiation Regulations 1999 should be adhered to
- Someone within the practice should be appointed as the radiation protection supervisor (RPS)
- Every practice should appoint a radiation protection advisor (RPA)
- Local rules should be available for the practice
- A system of work should be devised for the individual practice
- A controlled area is the room in which the X-ray machine is being used
- The supervised area surrounds the controlled area
- Dose limits ensure that the dose received by personnel is kept to a minimum

Practical Veterinary Diagnostic Imaging, Second Edition. Suzanne Easton.
© 2012 John Wiley & Sons, Ltd. Published 2012 by Blackwell Publishing Ltd.

- Monitoring badges record the amount of doses received by an individual
- There are two types of monitoring devices: a film badge and a thermoluminescent dosimeter
- Lead shielding should be worn or used if it is essential for an individual to remain in the controlled area during an exposure
- Quality assurance involves both the X-ray machine and the processor
- Quality assurance monitors changes to the equipment that may reduce radiation safety

Introduction

Radiation safety should be remembered at all times when carrying out radiographic examinations. Adherence to the guidelines would ensure maximum safety for all personnel involved in diagnostic radiography. The guidelines are not designed to cause difficulties for the practitioner attempting to adhere to them but to ensure their safety and protection. The biggest factor in radiation safety is distance. The greater the distance from the primary beam to an individual, the safer the situation.

The effects of ionising radiation on the body

Ionising radiation can originate from the X-ray tube or in the form of gamma rays. This radiation damages cells and is not selective of cell type. The effects are more obvious in the immature or rapidly dividing cells. The amount of cell damage is determined by the amount of dose, the type of cell and its maturity. If the cell is still being formed when the dose is received, then the DNA may mutate. Later in the cell cycle, repair may occur.

Biological effects	**Heat, excitation and ionisation**
Cellular effects	**Somatic, carcinogenic and mutation**

The basics to remember

Radiation protection has three basic principles that should be adhered to at all times. If these principles are always remembered, then radiation safety will be maintained. The overall principle is known as the ALARA principle, which should be adhered to at all times. ALARA stands for As Low As Reasonably Achievable and can be maintained if the basics principles are remembered:

> 1 **No dose limit should be exceeded.**
> 2 **Exposure to personnel should be kept to a minimum.**
> 3 **Unnecessary procedures should not be performed.**

Ionising Radiation Regulations 1999

The law governing the use of radiation was revised in 1999/2000 and is given in full in the document entitled 'The Ionising Radiation Regulations 1999'. This gives all the information needed when using a source of radiation. The law also gives a number of regulations regarding maximum dose and control within the X-ray room.

All exposures used should be recorded along with patient details and stored with the machine. If there is no option but to manually restrain a patient, then the holder must be documented with the exposures used.

There is also a publication especially for veterinary use of radiation entitled 'Guidance Notes for the Protection of Persons against Ionising Radiations arising from Veterinary Use'. This has specific guidelines for the veterinary practice.

Radiation safety in the veterinary practice

If the suggestions laid out by the regulations are followed, then the safety of patients and personnel is maximised.

To maintain the safety levels necessary, practices must carry out the following:

1 The practice will need to appoint a Radiation Protection Supervisor (RPS). This is someone from within the practice who ensures that all the work is carried out safely.
2 A Radiation Protection Advisor (RPA) from outside the practice will be appointed. This person will help set up the working practices within the practice and the local rules.

Local rules

The local rules vary from one practice to another, but should ensure the following:

- No animal is manually restrained.
- No unnecessary personnel stays in the room during exposure.

- Suitable protection is used.
- Predetermined guidelines for pregnant members of staff.
- Minimum age of 16 for trainee staff.
- Areas within the practice are classified.
- Guidelines for the implementation of warning signs during exposure.

System of work

Details of this are prepared by the RPA and the RPS. This includes the local rules. These should be displayed where everyone can read them at any time. This is the legal responsibility of the RPS.

They should state the following:

- The name of the RPS.
- A description of the restricted areas.
- Details of access restriction.
- Details of working practices.
- Details of any plans should an incident occur.

RPA	**Radiation Protection Advisor**
RPS	**Radiation Protection Supervisor**
Local rules	**Guidelines specific to the practice**
System of work	**Includes local rules and gives details of the area classification and the names of the RPA, RPS and any other important information related to radiation safety**

Classifying the areas around an X-ray machine

These areas are defined by the RPA and maintained by the RPS when X-rays are being taken.

Controlled area

A controlled area is the room in which the X-ray machine is positioned. The area is so designated when the amount of dose within the area exceeds 7.5 mSv/h. People who enter this area should be identified and monitored, with records kept of all the readings recorded from their monitoring devices.

The controlled area should have brick walls (stud walls do not provide adequate safety) and the room should be large enough to allow two people to stand at least 2 m from the tube. A warning sign with the radiation trefoil in black on a yellow background should be placed at the entrance of the room and the number of people within the classified area kept to a minimum. An indication of when an exposure is being made is also compulsory either as a beep on the machine or a light outside the room (Figure 14.1).

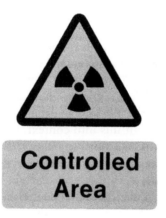

Figure 14.1   Example of a warning sign to be used outside of a controlled area.

Supervised area

A supervised area surrounds the controlled area. This is any area that exceeds 1/10 of the recommended dose limit; therefore, control of personnel entering this area needs to be monitored.

Dose limits

Dose levels are the amount of radiation received by an individual over a set period of time. These dose levels are controlled by legislation. They are designed to ensure that the dose received by personnel is kept to a minimum. If you ever need an X-ray yourself, you become a member of the general public at this point and not classified/trainee. You should not wear your monitoring device. The levels for classified personnel are designed to include not only people using diagnostic X-rays, but also those exposed to radiation in power stations and other industrial settings. These levels are decreasing each time the legislation is reviewed.

All doses must be recorded and transferred when staff moves practices. The doses should be recorded using either a film badge or thermoluminescent dosimeter (TLD).

Records of the exposures used for each case must also be kept. Such records should be kept with the machine used or with the radiograph produced. The kV, mAs and distance used along with the film type and examination should always be recorded. It is also important to record details of any personnel who remained in the room during the exposure. If the machine is fitted with a dose area product (DPA) meter, then the reading from this should be documented for each examination.

Monitoring devices

Monitoring devices are not compulsory, but advisable. The use of these ensures that personnel receive the minimum dose and anything that is received above this is known about. It also ensures that the maximum does limits are not exceeded. The usual annual dose received by monitored personnel using diagnostic X-rays is approximately 2 mSv. To put this into context, background radiation in the United Kingdom is 1–2 mSv.

The readings from dosimeters are cumulative and are maintained throughout the individual's career. Monitoring badges should not be shared by individuals and should be worn under protective clothing. This will give an accurate indication of the dose received by the body (rather than the dose received by the apron).

There are a number of different monitoring devices:

Film badge

A small film is placed in a plastic container. A number of different ports have varying thicknesses and types of metal. When the film is developed, the degree of blackening on the film and the regions that are blackened will determine the dose received. The films are sent away for analysis and can only be used once, making them expensive (Figure 14.2).

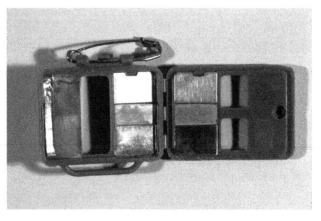

Figure 14.2   Open film badge.

Thermoluminescent dosimeter

The thermoluminescent dosimeter is of similar size to the film badge. It contains crystals of lithium fluoride, which has a similar density to soft tissues. After the dosimeter has been worn and possibly irradiated, it is heated, and the amount of light emitted is compared to a standard, known radiation dose. The dose received can then be calculated. This type of monitor can be reused (Figure 14.3).

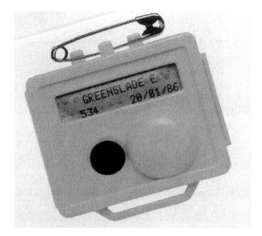

Figure 14.3   Thermoluminescent dosimeter.

Lead shielding

If there is no alternative and personnel must remain in the room whilst an exposure is being made, lead protection must be used. This is usually in the form of a lead apron or a lead-lined screen. These contain a certain amount of lead and give protection against scattered radiation. Scattered radiation protection is measured in lead equivalent and is usually 0.5 mm for a lead apron. Lead shielding is only effective against scattered radiation. The energy levels in the primary beam are high enough to allow penetration through the lead. Scatter radiation has low energy levels; so it is absorbed by the lead.

Monitoring devices should be worn under the apron so that the dose received by the individual is accurately monitored. Lead aprons need to be checked from time to time for cracks that may reduce the protection received from the apron. Visual inspection will reveal any holes forming and even fairly small holes can be detected in this way.

In equine radiography, if a film holder is used or the film is held during examination of the stifle, then lead gloves must be used by the individual as well as a lead apron.

All protection needs to be stored carefully. Folding is not advised as this may cause cracks or splits in the lead rubber. The ideal way to store an apron is hung up with no restrictions or compression on any part of the apron. Sheets of lead, gloves or sleeves should also be stored flat to prevent cracks from appearing (Figure 14.4).

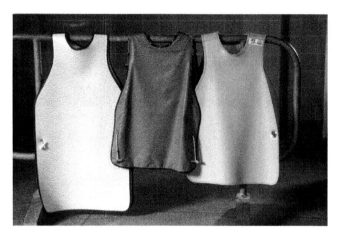

Figure 14.4   Lead shielding.

Quality assurance

Quality assurance (QA) forms an important part of the maintenance of a radiographic service and is an essential part of radiation protection. If QA is not carried out, there will be no baseline from which to determine any problems that may be present with the machine. Quality assurance covers both the X-ray machine and the processor. Both have an influence on the quality of radiographs being produced. Problems may occur with a machine, and over time exposure factors are increased or altered to accommodate the changes. This is not a good practice, and the problem can be detected through QA before exposure factors are altered. For consistency, one individual should carry out QA.

X-ray machine

Quality assurance can be carried out in practice on a routine basis as part of the annual service all equipment should receive. With the X-ray tube, this should include checks on the filtration, the accuracy of the timer and the correspondence between the kV_p selected and what the tube is actually delivering. Specialist equipment is needed for these checks, which may be beyond the financial resources and technical abilities of the individual practice.

Light-beam diaphragm checks

The accuracy of the light-beam diaphragm can be checked within the practice very easily and can rectify disputes over collimation practice. The primary beam is collimated to a square about 5 cm smaller than the cassette. Paper clips are unwound and placed on the corners of the visible collimation. Using a low exposure, the film is exposed. This is then processed. On viewing, the edge of the collimation should be at the same place as the paper clips. Any variation will demonstrate the inaccuracy of the collimators.

Processor

The QA necessary on a processor is varied, but should be carried out routinely – at least monthly. The rollers and tanks should be thoroughly washed with fresh running water. The temperature of the wash water and the developer should be checked, as these will influence the activity of the processing chemistry and the quality of the resultant image. Replenishment should be ongoing, as tired chemistry will reduce the effectiveness of the developing and fixing agents. Sensitometry and densitometry should be carried out to ensure the maintenance of constant processing conditions.

Further reading

BVA (2002) Guidance Notes for the Safe Use of Ionising Radiations in Veterinary Practice, BVA.
This publication provides a clear summary of the radiation regulations with key reference to veterinary practice.

Revision questions

1 Give two forms of ionising radiation.

2 How will ionising radiation affect cells?

3 What will be affected by the genetic effects of radiation?

4 What are the three basic principles associated with decreasing radiation exposure?

5 Which guidelines should be followed?

6 What is the RPA?

7 Give three points that the local rules should include.

8 Who devises the system of work?

(continued)

9 What type of walls should a controlled area have?

10 Where is the supervised area?

11 What is the minimum age of a classified worker?

12 How does a film badge record the dose received?

13 How does a TLD work?

14 List three QA tests or procedures that can be carried out easily by a practice.

Chapter 15

Radiography Principles

Chapter contents

General principles
Restraint
Positioning aids
Markers and legends
Assessing the radiograph
Terminology
BVA/KC hip dysplasia and elbow scoring scheme
Further reading

Key points

- Examinations should be clinically indicated and make a difference to the management of the patient
- Standard projections should be produced where possible
- Restraint should be employed to ensure diagnostic images are obtained
- As well as chemical restraint, positioning aids can be used to produce carefully positioned diagnostic images
- All images should be clearly marked with patient identification and anatomical markers
- Images should be assessed following clear, consistent criteria

Introduction

Once a full understanding of how an X-ray machine works and how manipulation of exposure factors influence the final radiograph is gained, then positioning will take on more meaning and can be used to produce a diagnostic and visually pleasing image. Through the use of a personal routine, the process of taking a radiograph can be efficient without missing any of the vital stages that may have a detrimental

Practical Veterinary Diagnostic Imaging, Second Edition. Suzanne Easton.
© 2012 John Wiley & Sons, Ltd. Published 2012 by Blackwell Publishing Ltd.

effect of the image quality. At all times radiation safety must take priority over all other considerations.

General principles

To ensure maximum benefit from accurate positioning, the following principles should be followed:

- Only films that are clinically indicated should be taken. 'For completeness', 'because the owner thinks ...' or 'because it would be nice' are not acceptable reasons for a radiograph.
- Radiation safety guidelines must be adhered to at all times.
- Standard projections should always be taken in the first instance. If this is not done, interpretation is more difficult and accurate diagnoses may not be possible.
- Standard projections are always a pair of projections at 90° to each other. This prevents pathology from being missed, either by other structures overlying or the pathology only being visible in one projection.
- Careful positioning centring and collimation should be maintained at all times.
- If a horizontal beam is being used, consideration should be given to the path of the primary beam after it has passed through the animal.
- If the positioning will compromise the animal's condition, careful consideration should be given to the outcome of performing the investigation.
- Careful indexing and cross referencing should be in place so that films can be easily found and repeats are not performed as films are 'lost'.

Restraint

To prevent the production of low quality or non-diagnostic images, some means of restraint is usually necessary. At no time should an animal be held. Regardless of how ill the animal is, some means of chemical sedation or aids for restraint with patience, are all that are needed with patience to get a diagnostic radiograph. Attempting radiographs with no sedation at all may result in a non-diagnostic image and a breakdown in the radiation safety practices being employed. This should be avoided at all times.

Examination of the spine, skull, pharynx, some contrast examinations, hip examinations and most fracture investigations should not be carried out unless the animal is anaesthetised. Even with heavy sedation, positioning will not be accurate as there will still be some muscle tone causing rotation and possible misinterpretation.

Positioning aids

As well as chemical restraint, positioning aids can be used to produce carefully positioned diagnostic images. These aids should be available for all examinations. Care must be taken to prevent artefacts from the aids being seen on the radiographs. Positioning aids can also be a source of cross-infection and contamination, so care must be taken to keep them clean. The radio-opacity of all aids should be known before use to prevent repeat radiographs from artefacts. Examples are:

- Radiolucent foam or plastic troughs for dorso-ventral or ventro-dorsal projections.
- A selection of radiolucent foam wedges and blocks: These should be in a variety of shapes and sizes. The range should include 45° wedges, square blocks and strips of foam. These should be washed after any use and contact with contrast medium.
- A selection of long floppy sandbags: These should not be placed in the primary beam, as they will be seen on the radiograph.
- Hobbles or bandages: These can be used to tie limbs out of the way or to hold the mouth open during examination of the bullae. These should not be used unless the animal is anaesthetised.
- Skull box: This is a box with graduated holes to accommodate bar for holding the patient in position when imaging the bullae or frontal sinuses.
- Positioning blocks and film holders are essential for equine examinations.
- A rope head collar is needed to prevent artefacts from being seen when imaging the equine head.

Markers and legends

All films should have anatomical markers that indicate the limb, the recumbency or the side of the patient. Markers should be placed so that they fall just outside the primary beam. This ensures that they are not over the region of interest but are seen in the scatter at the edges of the image. In equine work, the lateral aspect of the distal extremities should be marked so that lesions can be orientated. If films are part of a contrast examination, preliminary films and timed films should be marked. Markers come in a number of forms. The most common are metal clips or plastic tablets with the lead letters or markers embedded in the plastic. Whichever type is used, they will provide a permanent mark on the film

All radiographs should have a permanent mark of the animals and owner's names and the date of examination. This can be in the form of

X-Rite tape or through a marker that exposes the film with the details after exposure to the X-rays but before processing. This is known as an actinic marker. It is simple to use and provides a readable and permanent means of identification.

Pre- and post-exposure labelling

All radiographs should be labelled prior to processing. This can be either during the exposure using X-Rite tape or after exposure using an actinic light marker.

X-Rite tape is a special tape that when the details are written on it will allow them to be seen on the radiograph after processing. The tape strip must be in or close to the primary beam to be effective.

An actinic light marker will photograph the patient details onto the film after exposure but prior to processing. This uses a small light source to photograph the patient details onto the film. An area must be screened off on the film to allow this marker to be effective.

All films should have a minimum of the date and the patient details. A label added after processing is likely to fall off over time or be rubbed of the film.

Assessing the radiograph

When assessing a radiograph, the following points must always be considered:

- Identification present and correct.
- Markers and legends visible and correct.
- Area under examination shown.
- Correct projection taken.
- Suitable exposure factors used for area under examination.
- Adequate contrast, density and sharpness.
- Collimation visible but not too tight.
- Artefacts.
- Any anatomical variants or gross pathology present that may alter exposure factors.
- Good image quality.
- Need for further projections or repeats.

Terminology

All X-rays are described in terms of the path of the X-ray beam through the animal towards the film (Figures 15.1 and 15.2).

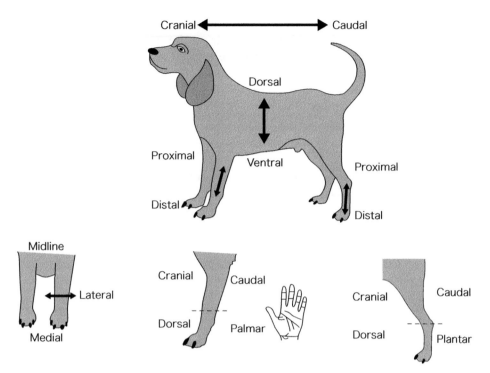

Figure 15.1   Terminology associated with small animal radiography.

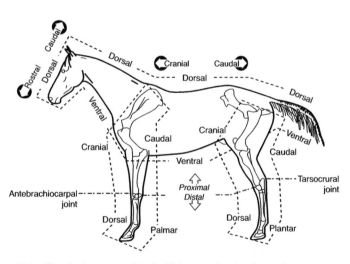

Figure 15.2   Terminology associated with large animal radiography.

It may also tell you how the animal was lying on the table. If an animal was lying with its right side on the table, it is a right lateral recumbent film. This film will be marked as a 'right' lateral. Some projections are at an angle and this will also be added into the description of the projection (Table 15.1). This is done most commonly in equine examinations.

Table 15.1   Terminology and abbreviations used in radiography.

Full description	Abbreviation	Direction of X-ray beam or description or area
Left	L	
Right	R	
Dorsal	D	Front of lower limbs or top of main trunk
Ventral	V	Underside of animal
Cranial	Cr	Towards the head
Caudal	Cd	Towards the tail
Rostral	R	Towards the nose
Medial	M	Inside of leg
Lateral	L	Outside edge of legs
Proximal	Pr	The higher end of an extremity or bone
Distal	Di	The part of a bone or limb furthest from the main body
Palmar	Pa or P	Back edge of the lower fore limb
Plantar	Pl	Back edge of the lower hind limb
Oblique	O	
Lesion Orientated Oblique	LOO	An oblique projection to skyline a lesion

BVA/KC hip dysplasia and elbow scoring scheme

For both of these schemes, set protocols should be followed. These are outlined below. Every animal undergoing these procedures must be over the age of one year and must have a kennel club certificate. Once taken, the radiographs and relevant paperwork should be sent to BVA for scoring. Each breed has a specific score, and the aim of the scheme is to minimise dysplasia by not breeding from animals with poor hips:

1 All animals must be over 1 year of age and have a kennel club certificate.

2 The dog should be anaesthetised and placed in dorsal recumbency with the hind limbs extended so that the femora are parallel to the table top.

3 The stifles should be rotated inwards and a tie placed just above them to hold them in place. Sandbags and troughs may be needed to obtain good positioning.

4 The Kennel Club registration number, the date and a left or right marker must be radiographed onto the film before processing. Nothing should be added to the film after processing.

5 The films are then sent away for scoring after which a written report will be sent to the veterinary surgeon and the owner.

Further reading

Norris, S. (2011) Canine hip dysplsia – a review. *Veterinary Nursing Journal* 26, 46–48.
Easton, S. (2002) Surface landmarks: their identification and use. *Veterinary Nursing* 17(5), 172–174.
Both of these articles provide further information on the areas introduced in this chapter.

Revision questions

1 Identify three methods of patient restraint.

2 What type of restraint should not be used with sedated or conscious patients?

3 List three criteria for assessing an image.

4 What does cranial, caudal, ventral and dorsal denote?

5 What are the positioning and image criteria for a kennel club hip score submission?

Chapter 16

Contrast Media

Chapter contents

Negative contrast medium
Positive contrast medium
Contrast examination procedures
Myelography
Other contrast examinations
Further reading

Key points

- Negative contrast medium can be air, oxygen, carbon monoxide or nitrous oxide
- It will appear black on radiographs
- Barium sulphate should not be given to anaesthetised or heavily sedated animals as inhalation may occur
- In double contrast studies, positive contrast must always be administered before negative contrast
- Positive contrast medium always has a high atomic number
- Positive contrast medium will appear white on radiographs
- Barium sulphate is used for investigation of the alimentary tract
- It is a white chalky powder that is mixed with water to give a liquid suspension
- Barium is insoluble
- Barium is not acted upon by digestive enzymes
- Water-soluble iodine compounds are used for all other types of contrast examinations
- They are in the form of clear liquids
- The concentration is described in milligrams of iodine per millilitre of medium
- Water-soluble contrast medium is either ionic or non-ionic
- Non-ionic contrast medium is safe to use in all areas, but is more expensive
- Ionic contrast medium has a high osmolarity and should not be used for myelography or examination of very weak patients

Practical Veterinary Diagnostic Imaging, Second Edition. Suzanne Easton.
© 2012 John Wiley & Sons, Ltd. Published 2012 by Blackwell Publishing Ltd.

- A protocol for each examination should be followed to ensure diagnostic examinations
- All contrast must be removed from the X-ray table and equipment after use to prevent artefacts from being seen on radiographs

Introduction

Contrast medium can be used to enhance structures that are not normally seen on plain radiography in detail or to outline cavities that may not be visible on plain radiographs. Contrast medium is divided into two distinct categories: positive and negative. Negative is usually air. This will appear black on radiographs. Positive contrast mediums include barium and iodine-based compounds. Both of these will appear white on radiographs. Examinations using contrast medium should follow protocols so that vital information or projections are not excluded.

Negative contrast medium

Negative contrast medium is usually in the form of air, but can be oxygen, carbon dioxide or nitrous oxide. Air is the negative contrast medium of choice as it is cheap and readily available. Air will appear black on radiographs.

Air can be used in conjunction with positive contrast media to give a double contrast study. Positive contrast can be used to coat any hollow structure. Air is then used to distend the structure. Air should be introduced after the positive contrast medium, otherwise bubbles and uneven coating may occur. The positive contrast will cling to the lining and the air will highlight defects. This method can be used in cystography and barium enema studies.

Positive contrast medium

All positive contrast media are selected because they have a high atomic number. This increases the absorption of X-rays and will appear white on radiographs. The two types available are barium sulphate based and a water-soluble iodine compound.

Barium sulphate

This contrast medium is used to outline the alimentary tract. It is a white chalky powder that is mixed with water to produce a liquid suspension or a paste. It may be supplied as a ready-made colloidal suspension, although this is not ideal if the use of the medium is limited in practice as once opened it is difficult to store (Table 16.1).

Table 16.1 Barium sulphate preparations.

Presentation	Proprietary name	Manufacturer
Powder	Micropaque HD	Nicholas
	Baritop Plus	Bioglan
	E-Z-Paque	Henleys
Suspension	Baritop 100	Bioglan
	Micropaque standard	Nicholas

Barium is completely insoluble and is not acted upon by digestive enzymes or absorbed by the intestine. Care should be taken however if it leaks into the peritoneum or is inhaled as it may result in granulomatous adhesions or aspiration pneumonia. The barium may cause faeces to appear white and cause constipation.

Iodine compounds

Iodine compounds used for contrast examinations are all water-soluble and appear as clear liquids. The water-soluble iodine compounds are usually used for all examinations other than those of the alimentary tract. They are not usually used for the alimentary tract unless perforation is suspected, as they are bitter to the taste, making it difficult to introduce them to conscious animals and do not give good contrast when compared with barium sulphate. They are usually more viscous than water and are very sticky. As they are water-soluble they can be injected directly into the vascular system. The contrast medium is excreted by the kidneys soon after injection and can therefore be used for examinations of the kidneys, ureters and bladder.

Water-soluble iodine compounds come in varying concentrations. The concentration is expressed as the amount of iodine per millilitre of medium. As an example, Conray 420 will contain 420 mg of iodine in every millilitre. Depending on the area under examination, a suitable concentration should be selected. This decision should take into consideration the amount of dilution that will occur after introduction (Table 16.2).

> **Concentration of water-soluble iodine compounds: milligrams of iodine per millilitre of medium**

Water-soluble contrast medium falls into two categories: ionic and non-ionic. Ionic contrast medium can cause adverse reactions

Table 16.2 Water-soluble iodine preparations.

Presentation	Ionic/non-ionic	Proprietary name	Concentration (mg I/mL)	Manufacturer	Uses
Sodium iothalamate	Ionic	Conray 420	420	Mallinkrodt	IVUs angiography
Sodium/meglumine iothalamate	Ionic	Conray 280	280	Mallinkrodt	IVUs
Sodium/meglumine diatrozoate	Ionic	Urografin 150	150	Schering	Sinography, fistulography, bladder studies
Iopamidol	Non-ionic	Niopam 300/370	300/370	E Merck	All contrast studies except myelography
Iohexol	Non-ionic	Omnipaque 240/300/350	240/300/350	Nycomed Amersham	All examinations

including vomiting, irritation and anaphylaxis. These reactions are due to the high osmolar pressure of the contrast medium and the toxicity of the contrast medium on normal body fluids. These contrast mediums should only be used for introduction into cavities such as the bladder or intravenously in healthy patients.

If the patient is unwell or is undergoing myelography, more expensive non-ionic contrast mediums should be used. These have a lower osmolality and cause fewer side effects. Care should be taken to ensure that they are recommended for use during myelography.

Contrast examination procedures

To ensure maximum benefit from the expensive and time-consuming examinations, a number of principles need to be remembered:

- Proper preparation of the patient should be ensured.
- Adequate sedation or anaesthesia should be administered.
- Preliminary radiographs should always be taken before the introduction of contrast medium. This will ensure suitable exposure factors are used and will demonstrate any abnormalities that may not be visible after the contrast medium has been introduced.
- Adequate contrast medium of a suitable concentration should be given.
- Any spillage should be removed immediately to prevent artefacts.
- Positioning and collimation should be accurate.

Gastrointestinal tract

Examination	**Barium swallow**
Use of examination	Used to outline the oesophagus
Indications	Regurgitation
	Retching/dysphagia
	Suspicion of foreign bodies
Patient preparation	None required
Sedation	Mild sedation if essential
	Barium should not be administered if the animal is
	heavily sedated or anaesthetised
Dose	Liquid barium sulphate suspension
	Dogs: 5–20-mL liquid depending on size
	Cats: Up to 5 mL of liquid depending on size
	Or a small quantity of paste or barium mixed
	with food
	Do not use food if you want to follow the barium
	through from the stomach

Examination	**Barium swallow**
Administration of contrast medium	Use a syringe in the corner of the mouth or allow the food or barium paste to be eaten Avoid spillage
Radiographic technique	• Plain lateral radiograph of the thorax before giving the barium • Thorax immediately after administration

Examination	**Barium meal and/or follow through**
Use of examination	To outline the stomach and duodenum
Indications	Vomiting
Patient preparation	No food for 12 hours No water for 2 hours
Sedation	Moderate sedation to allow multiple radiographic views to be taken
Dose	Liquid barium sulphate suspension *Dogs*: 1–3 mL per kilogram body weight *Cats and very small dogs*: 2–5 mL per kilogram body weight
Administration of contrast medium	By mouth with a syringe (some animals may drink the barium) Using a stomach tube. This ensures that no inhalation takes place and that the barium is introduced quickly in one dose

Radiographic technique	• Preliminary plain lateral and ventro-dorsal films of the abdomen should be taken
	• If fluoroscopy is available, this can be used to watch the movement of the stomach
	• Four views of the stomach should be taken immediately after administration:
	    Right lateral recumbency
	    Ventro-dorsal
	    Left lateral recumbency
	    Dorso-ventral
	    This will ensure that all areas of the stomach are demonstrated
	• Take ventro-dorsal and right lateral recumbency films, centred for the abdomen every 30 minutes until the stomach has emptied completely
	• To demonstrate the small intestine, radiographs should be taken every hour after the stomach is empty (Figure 16.1)

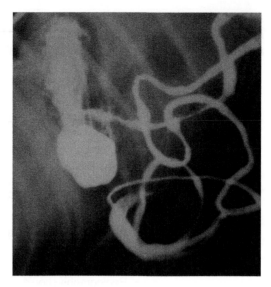

Figure 16.1   Barium follow-through.

Examination	**Barium enema**
Use of examination	Used to demonstrate large bowel if proctoscopy is not available
Indications	Melaena
	Chronic diarrhoea
	Tenesmus
Patient preparation	The animal should be fed a low residue diet for 3 days
	A non-irritant enema should be administered 2–3 hours before the examination to ensure that the bowel is empty
Sedation	General anaesthesia or very heavy sedation
Dose	Dilute liquid barium mixed fifty-fifty with warm water
	Approximately 10 mL per kilogram body weight
Administration of contrast medium	A bag containing the contrast medium and water should be hung from a drip stand
	A Foley catheter should be inserted into the rectum, attached to a rubber tube with a method of controlling the flow of barium (clamp is ideal)
	Barium should be allowed to flow slowly into the rectum by gravity

Examination ***Radiographic*** ***technique***	**Barium enema**
	• Ventro-dorsal and right lateral recumbency plain films of the abdomen should be taken
	• Radiographs of the bowel should be taken after introduction of the barium in:
	  Right lateral recumbency
	  Left lateral recumbency
	  Ventro-dorsal
	• kV should be increased to penetrate the edges of the barium
	• If a double contrast enema is required, the barium should be removed from the colon, again by gravity
	• Air should be introduced into the colon to make the barium cling to the mucosa and highlight any defects in the surface
	• Radiographs should be repeated with the kV reduced to prevent overexposure

Genito-urinary tract

Examination	**Intravenous urography**
Use of examination	Used to demonstrate the function and anatomy of the kidneys and ureters
Indications	Incontinence Persistent haematuria Pyelonephritis Trauma
Patient preparation	Food should be removed for 12 hours and water for 2 hours before examination A cleansing enema should be given before the study as faeces in the colon may overlay the kidneys and ureters The bladder should be emptied
Sedation	General anaesthesia is essential to prevent movement during the examination
Dose	*Conray 420*: 1 mL per kilogram body weight *Conray 280*: 2 mL per kilogram body weight
Administration of ***contrast medium***	Rapid intravenous injection as a bolus *Or* a rapid drip infusion if a low concentration of iodine is being used (Urografin 150)

Examination
Radiographic
technique

Intravenous urography
- Plain right lateral recumbency and ventro-dorsal films centred on the umbilicus should be taken before introduction of the contrast
- From the end of injection
- Immediate ventro-dorsal film at the level of the umbilicus
- 5-min ventro-dorsal film at the level of the umbilicus
- 10-min right lateral recumbency film at the level of the umbilicus
- 15-min right lateral recumbency film centred at the level of the bladder neck
- More radiographs may be necessary if abnormalities are detected or excretion is slow (Figure 16.2)

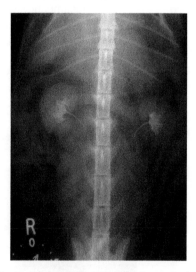

Figure 16.2 Five-minute VD abdomen image from an intravenous urography in a cat.

Examination
Use of examination
Indications

Urethrogram – male
To demonstrate the bladder, urethra and prostate
Incontinence – may be used in conjunction with an IVU
Dysuria
Persistent haematuria
Trauma
Position of bladder

Examination	**Urethrogram – male**
Patient preparation	A cleansing enema is useful, but not essential
Sedation	General anaesthesia is recommended but not essential
Dose	Urografin 150 or more concentrated contrast, diluted with sterile water
	Approximately 2 mL per kilogram
Administration of contrast medium	A small Foley catheter is introduced into the penile urethra and the cuff inflated to prevent the escape of the contrast medium
	The Foley catheter should be flushed with contrast before insertion to prevent the introduction of air bubbles
	Hands and forearms should be protected with lead gloves or sheets
Radiographic technique	• A plain film should be taken in right lateral recumbency, centred for the bladder neck and collimated to include the whole urethra
	• The bladder should then be catheterised and emptied
	• The animal should be repositioned as before
	• The contrast should be injected and the film exposed during the injection (Figure 16.3)

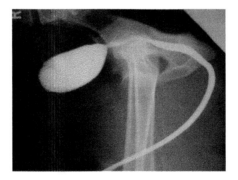

Figure 16.3   Male retrograde urethrogram.

Examination	**Urethrogram – female**
Use of examination	To demonstrate the bladder, urethra and vagina – may be used in conjunction with an IVU
Indications	Incontinence
	Dysuria
	Persistent haematuria
	Trauma
	Position of bladder

Examination	**Urethrogram – female**
Patient preparation	A cleansing enema is useful, but not essential
Sedation	General anaesthesia is essential
Dose	Urografin 150 or more concentrated contrast, diluted with sterile water
	Approximately 1 mL per kilogram to fill the vagina and urethra
Administration of contrast medium	A small Foley catheter is placed in the vestibule of the vagina and the cuff inflated to prevent the escape of the contrast medium. The catheter is held in place and placing Allis tissue forceps across the vulva prevents back flow of the contrast. This can stimulate the animal and adequate anaesthesia is essential
	The Foley catheter should be flushed with contrast before insertion to prevent the introduction of air bubbles
	Hands and forearms should be protected with lead gloves or sheets
	The contrast medium should be introduced in small increments, with the first film taken after 2/3 of the medium is introduced
	If the urethra is not full, then more contrast medium can be introduced
Radiographic technique	• A plain film should be taken in right lateral recumbency, centred for the bladder neck and collimated to include the whole urethra
	• The bladder should then be catheterised and emptied
	• The animal should be repositioned as before
	• The contrast should be injected and the film exposed during the injection
Examination	**Cystography**
Use of examination	Used to demonstrate the bladder
Indications	Dysuria
	Persistent haematuria
	Trauma
	Position of bladder
Patient preparation	A cleansing enema is useful, but not essential
Sedation	General anaesthesia is recommended but not essential

Examination	**Cystography**
Dose	*Pneumocystogram*: Air – 10 mL per kilogram body weight *or* until the bladder feels distended
	Positive contrast cystography: Urografin 150 – 10 mL per kilogram body weight
	Double contrast cystography: As for positive cystography, then remove contrast medium and replace with air
Administration of contrast medium	The bladder should be catheterised and urine removed
	The contrast medium or combination of contrast medium and air should be introduced slowly, and if resistance is felt, no further introduction should take place
Radiographic technique	• A plain film should be taken in right lateral recumbency, centred for the bladder neck
	• The bladder should then be catheterised and emptied
	• The animal should be repositioned as before
	• The contrast should be injected and the film exposed immediately after injection
	• For a pnemocystogram, the kV should be reduced

Myelography

Myelography is the introduction of positive contrast medium into the subarachnoid space around the spinal cord. The absence or deviation of the column of contrast medium surrounding the spinal cord will demonstrate lesions. Throughout this examination, speed is essential, as the contrast will be absorbed rapidly into the blood stream.

Indications	Spinal pain
	Paraplegia
	Quadriplegia
	Ataxia
	Trauma
Patient preparation	The contrast medium can be introduced through a cisternal or lumbar puncture. Whichever route is chosen, the area should be clipped and surgically cleaned to ensure sterility

Sedation	General anaesthesia essential
	Valium is often given just before the contrast is injected
Dose	0.3 mL per kilogram body weight of a non-ionic contrast medium up to 10 mL
	Hexabrix should *not* be used. Despite being of a low osmolarity, it contains Ioxaglate, a mono-acid dimer, which is ionic, and not a suitable contrast medium for use during myelography
Administration of contrast medium	*Cisternal puncture*: The head and shoulders should be raised 10° to prevent the contrast from flowing back into the ventricles of the brain. The head is flexed 90° to the neck. The spinal needle is inserted between the skull and the atlas until CSF drips from the needle. This should be collected in sterile containers for analysis. The contrast is injected slowly and the needle is then removed and the neck is extended
	Lumbar puncture: The spinal column is flexed by placing the front legs through the hind legs. This should not be done if there is any suspicion of instability of the spine. The needle is inserted at the level of the L4–5 or L5–6 junction. The hind legs will twitch as the needle passes through the spinal cord. Little or no CSF may appear and so a test radiograph will demonstrate the position of the needle and the contrast medium, before all of the contrast is introduced incorrectly. After introduction, the needle is removed and the spine is extended. The head should be raised to prevent the contrast from flowing into the ventricles of the brain
Radiographic technique	Preliminary lateral radiographs should be taken to demonstrate the area under suspicion
	A test radiograph may be necessary with a lumbar puncture. This should be in lateral recumbency centred over the needle
	Lateral projections should be taken of the spine starting at the injection site and moving with the contrast

Indications   Spinal pain

If the contrast does not flow, traction may be necessary. Tying a bandage around the maxilla, making a loop at the free end and hanging this with some heavy sandbags over the end of the table can achieve this

Once the contrast is at the area of interest, ventro-dorsal projections should be taken

In cases with suspected thoraco-lumbar lesions, following a lumbar puncture, the ventro-dorsal projection should be taken immediately (Figure 16.4)

If the cervical spine is involved, the endotracheal tube should be removed for the ventro-dorsal projection

Aftercare   The animal should be carefully monitored after myelography and the head should be kept raised until the animal has recovered fully from the anaesthesia

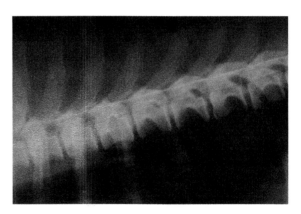

Figure 16.4   Thoracic myelogram.

Other contrast examinations

Arthrography

This examination will demonstrate the joint cavity and the articular surfaces. 1–1.5 mL of a non-ionic contrast medium is introduced into the joint and then radiographs are taken to demonstrate the position of the contrast. This is used mainly in the shoulder (Figure 16.5).

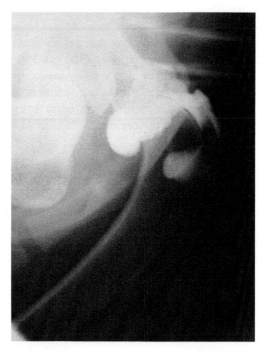

Figure 16.5   Shoulder arthrogram.

Portal venography

This is used to demonstrate the vessels within the liver. It will show whether the liver is receiving adequate blood flow and whether there are any anatomic abnormalities. It is the examination of choice for the diagnosis of a porto-systemic shunt.

At laparotomy, a vein in the jejunum is selected and a cannula inserted and tied in position. 5–10 mL of water-soluble iodine-based contrast medium is introduced as rapidly as possible and a radiograph, centred over the last rib is taken on completion of the injection.

Sinography and fistulography

This will demonstrate the tract of any discharging sinus and the presence of any foreign body present. Fistulography will demonstrate the presence and path of a fistula. A catheter is placed into the opening of the sinus tract or suspected fistula and secured in place. Contrast is then introduced, ensuring that there is no spillage or back flow. On completion of the injection or when resistance is experienced, a radiograph is taken.

Angiography and venography

Both of these examinations will demonstrate the vascular system. The best images are obtained when the catheter and contrast is placed directly into the vein or artery under investigation. A radiograph should be taken immediately after the termination of the injection. Some examinations may require films every 1–2 seconds to give adequate demonstration of the region.

Sialography

Used to demonstrate the salivary glands. Uses a very fine needle inserted into the salivary duct and the introduction of 0.5–1 mL of high concentration iodine-based contrast medium.

Dacryocystorhinogram

This examination will demonstrate the nasolacrimal duct in cats and dogs. Contrast is introduced through one of the puncta in the eye.

Arthrography	Joints
Portal venography	Hepatic portal veins
Sinogram	Sinus tract
Fistulogram	Fistula
Angiography	Arterial blood supply
Venogram	Venous blood supply
Sialogram	Salivary glands
Dacryocystorhinography	Nasolacrimal ducts

Further reading

Blundell, F. (2010) Practical notes on urinary tract radiography. *Veterinary Nursing Journal* 25(5), 29–32.
All contrast media come with a safety data sheet. This provides details of the chemical composition, safety advice and side effects. By reading this sheet, you can develop an understanding of the properties of contrast medium and the use of each type.
An excellent article providing more in-depth information on contrast studies of the urinary tract.

Revision questions

1 Give two reasons why air is the negative contrast agent of use.

2 What is a double contrast study?

3 Why should contrast medium be introduced before air?

(continued)

4 Describe a barium sulphate suspension.

5 Why should barium sulphate not be given to anaesthetised or heavily sedated animals?

6 How are iodine-based compounds introduced?

7 How much iodine does Urografin 150 contain?

8 Why should non-ionic contrast medium be used when available?

9 How much barium would you use in a barium swallow on a dog?

10 For a barium swallow, what radiographs would you take?

11 During a barium follow through, how often should radiographs be taken after the stomach has emptied?

12 Describe how barium should be administered for a barium enema.

13 List the patient preparation for an intravenous urogram.

14 What is the approximate dose of contrast medium needed for an intravenous urogram in a border collie?

15 How often should radiographs be taken during an intravenous urogram?

16 During an urethrogram, what protection should be used?

17 What will a double contrast cystogram demonstrate?

18 What type of contrast medium must be used for myelography?

19 What is the dose rate of contrast medium for myelography?

20 What is a sinogram?

Chapter 17

Small Animal Radiography Techniques

Chapter contents

Chest
Abdomen
Head and neck
Distal extremities
Shoulder
Pelvis
Spine
Small mammals
Birds
Reptiles

Chest

If lateral and ventro-dorsal (VD) or dorsal–ventral (DV) projections are to be taken, then the VD or DV should be taken before the lateral to ensure there is no misdiagnosis from positional collapse of the lungs.

A right lateral of the chest should be taken as the standard projection, but if there is suspicion of metastasis then an additional left lateral examination should be performed.

Right lateral recumbency

- Forelegs extended and sandbagged.
- Pad under sternum.
- Sandbag to hold hindlegs and neck.
- Centre midway between the sternum and the spine, level with the caudal border of the scapula.
- Collimate to include the front of the shoulder and the edge of the sternum (Figure 17.1).
- Expose on inspiration.

Practical Veterinary Diagnostic Imaging, Second Edition. Suzanne Easton.
© 2012 John Wiley & Sons, Ltd. Published 2012 by Blackwell Publishing Ltd.

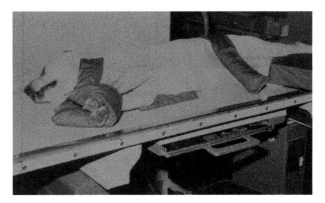

Figure 17.1   Positioning and restraint for a lateral chest.

DV chest

- Patient placed in dorsal recumbency.
- Chin supported on a pad.
- Sandbag over the neck.
- Forelegs pulled forward and adducted.
- Centre at the midline at the caudal prominences of the scapulae.
- Collimate to include the thoracic inlet and diaphragm (Figure 17.2).
- Expose on inspiration.

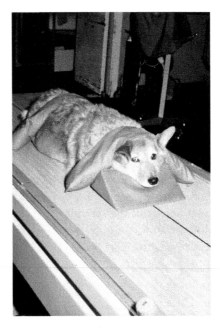

Figure 17.2   Positioning and restraint for a dorso-ventral chest.

VD chest

- Patient placed in ventral recumbency.
- Forelegs placed in a neutral position beside head and sandbagged.
- Centre at the midline at the mid-point of the sternum.
- Collimate to include the thoracic inlet and diaphragm (Figure 17.3).
- Expose on inspiration.

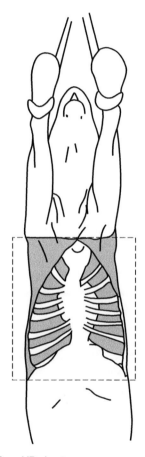

Figure 17.3 Positioning for a VD chest.

Abdomen

Right lateral recumbency

- Forelegs and hindlegs sandbagged.
- Pad under sternum.

- Centre at the 11th/12th intercostal space, just cranial to the last rib.
- Collimate to include diaphragm and symphysis (Figure 17.4).
- Expose just after expiration.

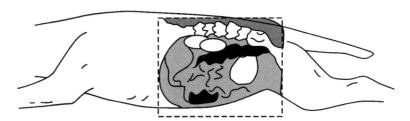

Figure 17.4   Positioning for a lateral view of the abdomen.

VD abdomen

- Patient placed in dorsal recumbency.
- Sandbags over carpi.
- Ensure that there is no rotation.
- Centre on the midline at the level of the umbilicus.
- Collimate to include diaphragm and symphysis (Figure 17.5).
- Expose just after expiration.

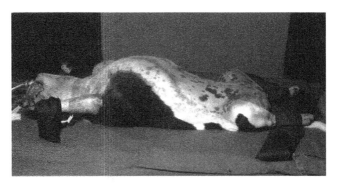

Figure 17.5   Positioning and restraint for a VD abdomen.

Head and neck

VD skull

- The patient is placed in dorsal recumbency and the neck is extended.

- A foam pad is placed under the neck to ensure that the hard palate is parallel to the cassette.
- Centring is on the midline to include the area of interest (entire skull or tympanic bulla area; Figure 17.6).

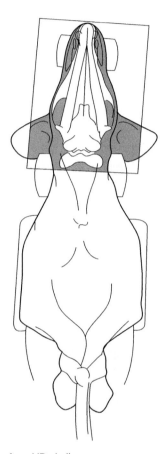

Figure 17.6   Positioning for a VD skull.

Lateral skull

- The patient is placed in lateral recumbency with the nose supported on a pad.
- A small pad is placed under the cervical spine to support the neck. The forelimbs are pulled towards the sternum to remove the limbs and soft tissue of the shoulder from the region of interest (Figure 17.7).
- Centring is to the area of interest.

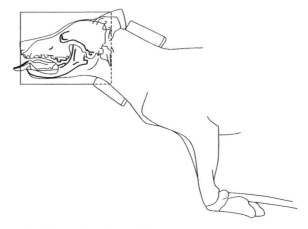

Figure 17.7   Positioning for a lateral skull.

Open mouth rostro-caudal view (tympanic bullae)

- The patient is placed on its back with the hard palate perpendicular to the cassette.
- The mouth is held wide open with tapes.
- The beam is parallel to the hard palate centred on the base of the tongue.
- The animal must have the endotracheal (ET) tube removed to demonstrate tympanic bulla adequately (Figure 17.8).

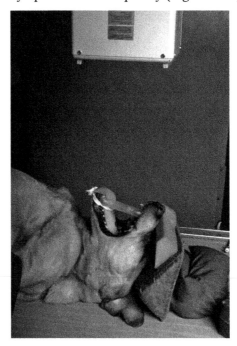

Figure 17.8   Positioning for an open mouth rostro-caudal view.

Rostro-caudal view (frontal sinuses)

- The patient is placed on its back with the hard palate perpendicular to the cassette.
- The beam is parallel to the hard palate centred on the middle of the nose.
- Collimation should include the area of the frontal sinuses.

Dorso-ventral intra-oral view (nasal chambers)

- The patient is supported in sternal recumbency with the neck extended.
- Place sandbag over the neck to prevent rotation.
- Place a non-screen film into the mouth, corner first as far into the mouth as possible.
- Centre the beam on a line midway between the external nares and a line joining the eyes.
- Ensure that an anatomical marker is included (Figure 17.9).

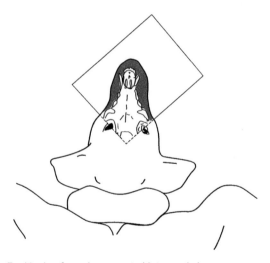

Figure 17.9   Positioning for a dorso-ventral intra-oral view.

Nasopharynx

- The patient is placed in lateral recumbency.
- A pad supports the skull in a true lateral position and a pad is placed under the neck.
- The legs are pulled caudally against the wall of the thorax.

- Centring is at the mid-cervical area to include the pharynx and thoracic inlet.
- The patient should be extubated prior to exposure.

Lateral oblique skull (temporo-mandibular joints, tympanic bullae)

- The patient is placed in lateral recumbency.
- The forelegs are pulled caudally against the chest wall and held with a sandbag.
- A pad is placed under the nose to raise it by approximately 30°. This will separate the temporo-mandibular joints (TMJs) or the bullae so that they can be seen more easily.
- Centring is directly over the uppermost TMJ or tympanic bulla and collimation should include a small area around the area of interest.
- The side nearest the film should be area under investigation.
- Both sides need to be imaged for comparison.

Oblique projection of the teeth

- The patient is placed in lateral recumbency.
- A gag is placed in the mouth to separate the mandible and the maxilla.
- The head is rotated slightly to remove the arcade nearest the tube away from the teeth under examination.
- The teeth under examination should be seen between the upper arcade nearest the tube and the teeth of the mandible or maxilla.
- Centring is on the last visible part of the tooth next to the gums.
- Collimation should demonstrate the arcade from the TMJ to the midline of the head.

Distal extremities

Medio-lateral

- The patient is placed with the side to be imaged nearest the cassette.
- The opposing limb is placed and supported on the flank (forelimbs pulled caudally, hindlimbs pulled cranially).
- The limb should be parallel with the cassette; a pad may be necessary to prevent rotation.

- Stifles and elbows should be flexed.
- Centring is at the level of the joint or mid-shaft.
- Collimation is to include a joint above and below the long bone or a small area above and below the joint under investigation (Figure 17.10).

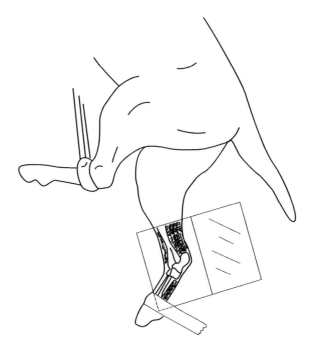

Figure 17.10   Medio-lateral of the right tarsus.

Dorso-palmar/plantar

Caudo-cranial

Horizontal beam

- The patient is placed with the limb under investigation uppermost.
- This limb is extended fully and supported with a pad so that it is parallel with the cassette.
- Centring is at the level of the joint or mid-shaft.
- Collimation is to include a joint above and below the long bone or a small area above and below the joint under investigation (Figure 17.11).

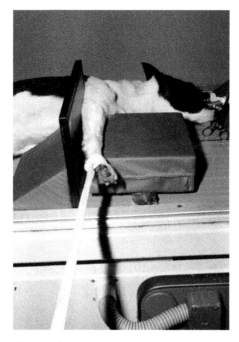

Figure 17.11   Positioning of an extremity using a horizontal beam.

Normal beam

- Patient is placed in sternal or dorsal recumbency so that the limb under investigation is parallel with the cassette.
- The opposing limb may need to be lifted to rotate the limb under investigation so that it is straight.
- Centring is at the level of the joint or mid-shaft.
- Collimation is to include a joint above and below the long bone or a small area above and below the joint under investigation (Figure 17.12).

Shoulder

Lateral

- The animal is placed in lateral recumbency with the limb to be radiographed nearest to the cassette.
- The head and neck are extended with sandbags.
- The upper limb is retracted and secured with sandbags.
- The limb under examination is drawn forward and ventrally.
- The beam is centred at the level of and caudal to the lateral tuberosity (Figure 17.13).

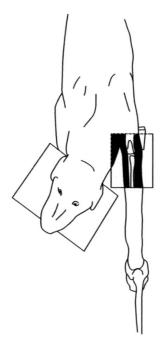

Figure 17.12   Positioning of the elbow.

Caudo-cranial

- The patient is placed on its back and supported with sandbags; the thorax may need to be rotated slightly.
- The affected limb is drawn cranially, fully extended and secured with a tie.
- The beam should be centred level with acromion process (Figure 17.14).

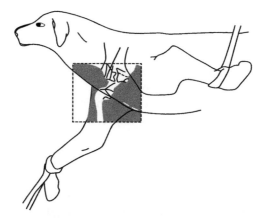

Figure 17.13   Positioning for the lateral of the shoulder.

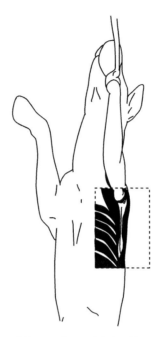

Figure 17.14   Positioning of the caudo-cranial shoulder.

Pelvis

Ventro-dorsal

- The patient is placed in dorsal recumbency ensuring that the body is straight.
- The hindlimbs are extended so that the femora are parallel and rotated medially.
- The hindlimbs are tied above the stifles with sandbags over the stifles and hocks to maintain position.
- The beam is centred at the level of the greater trochanter along the midline (Figure 17.15).

If the patient has a suspected fracture, a frog leg view may provide the necessary information.

The patient is placed on their backs and the legs are allowed to flop to the side to give the impression of a frog!

Lateral pelvis

- The patient is placed in lateral recumbency.
- Pads are placed between the hindlegs to ensure that the pelvis is not rotated.

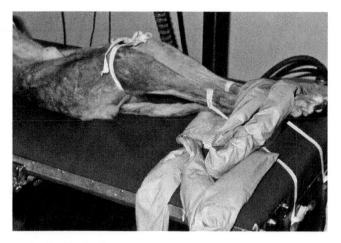

Figure 17.15 Positioning for a VD pelvis.

- The beam is centred over the greater trochanter and collimated to include the entire pelvis.

Spine

Lateral

- The patient should be placed in lateral recumbency.
- The spine should be supported with foam pads so that it is parallel with the tabletop.
- Pads should be placed under the sternum and between the limbs to prevent rotation.
- For the cervical spine, the forelimbs should be pulled caudally.
- The beam should be centred over the area of interest. If the entire spine is being examined, each image should overlap with the ones either side (Figure 17.16).

Lumbar sacral junction (lateral)

- This position has very specific positioning landmarks.
- The greater trochanter of the femur should be identified and the cranial part o the ilial wing.
- A line should be drawn between the two and centring should be on the middle of the imaginary line.

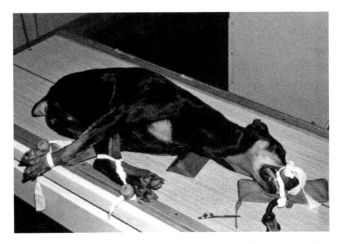

Figure 17.16   Positioning using sandbags and pads ready to centre for a spinal radiograph.

Ventro-dorsal

- The animal is placed on its back supported in a trough or with sandbags.
- The patient should be as straight as possible.
- The hindlegs should be extended to prevent rotation.
- The beam should be centred over the region of interest.

Small mammals

- All small mammals can be radiographed without a grid.
- Short exposure times can be used.
- A film giving high definition is ideal.
- The animal can be imaged in either lateral or dorsal recumbency; whichever keeps the animal the stillest.

Rabbits and guinea pigs

- For rabbits and guinea pigs, a trough and sandbags can be used in a similar way to imaging a small cat or dog.
- With adequate sedation they will remain still using only these restraints.

Mice, gerbils, hamsters

- Smaller mammals may need to be placed into a Perspex tube or a roll of exposed X-ray film to keep them contained and in position.

- Tape may be used to position the animal, although care must be taken to prevent them from struggling and causing further injuries (Figure 17.17).

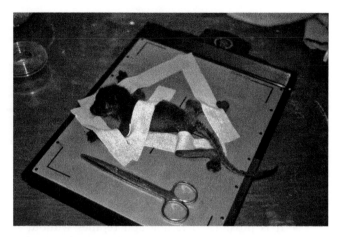

Figure 17.17   Imaging a small mammal.

Birds

Depending on the size of the bird, individual regions or the entire animal may be imaged.

Whole bird – ventro-dorsal

- If the whole bird is to be imaged, it should be placed in dorsal recumbency on the cassette.
- The wings should be extended to remove them from the body.
- The legs should be drawn caudally.
- The bird must be symmetrical to allow interpretation.
- The wings, neck and legs must be secured with tape.

Lateral

- The bird should be placed in lateral recumbency.
- The wings should be extended above the body and taped into position.
- The legs should be secured to improve imaging (if the legs are the area of interest) and to restrain the bird (Figure 17.18).

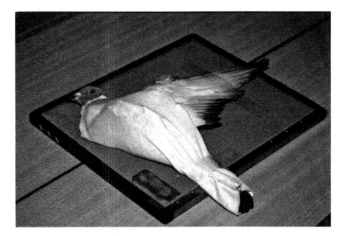

Figure 17.18 Positioning for a lateral projection of a bird.

Reptiles

- It is possible to radiograph reptiles without sedation if they are allowed to cool to room temperature and their heads are covered.
- No reptile will tolerate lateral recumbency and so a horizontal beam will be necessary if a lateral projection is required.
- Restraint can be achieved using a Perspex box or tube or through the use of tape. Restraint may not be necessary however for many of these animals.
- If the animal is too long to be fitted onto one film, multiple films can be used with overlap to ensure total coverage.

Chapter 18

Large Animal Radiography Techniques

Chapter contents

Foot
Fetlock
Metacarpus and metatarsus (cannon and splint)
Carpus
Elbow
Shoulder
Tarsus
Stifle
Head
Spine
Chest

Foot

Dorso-palmar of the pedal bone (DPr60°-PaDiO)

- The foot should be clean and trimmed, with the shoes removed.
- The frog should be packed to remove gas shadows. The packing material can be soap or play dough or other similar material.
- The film is placed in a film holder and the foot placed on top of this.
- The primary beam is centred below the coronary band on the midline of the foot with a downward angle of 60°.
- Collimation should include the edges of the hoof wall and the toe and heel of the foot (Figure 18.1).

Dorso-palmar of the navicular bone (DPr60°-PaDiO)

- The foot should be clean and trimmed, with the shoes removed.
- The frog should be packed to remove gas shadows.
- The film is placed in a film holder and the foot placed on top of this.

Practical Veterinary Diagnostic Imaging, Second Edition. Suzanne Easton.
© 2012 John Wiley & Sons, Ltd. Published 2012 by Blackwell Publishing Ltd.

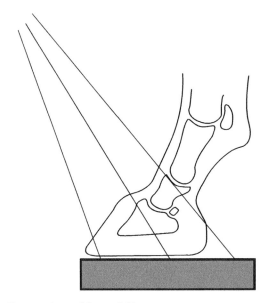

Figure 18.1   Dorso-palmar of the pedal bone.

- The primary beam is centred just above the coronary band on the midline of the foot with a downward angle of 60°.
- Collimation should be large enough to include all of the navicular bone.

Latero-medial of the pedal bone and navicular bone

- The foot is prepared as for the dorso-palmar (DP) projection.
- The foot is placed on a block to ensure that it is high enough off the ground.
- The horse should be bearing weight on the limb.
- The beam is projected parallel to the floor and centred at the level of the coronary band to include the heel and toe.
- Collimation should include the weight-bearing surface of the foot.

    If laminitis is suspected a lead strip, the top level with the coronary band should be placed down the midline of the hoof wall.

Palmaro-proximal–dorso-distal oblique of the navicular bone (Pa45Pr-DDiO)

- The foot is cleaned and trimmed, and the frog is packed to remove any gas shadows.
- The foot is placed on a film holder containing the film.

- The foot is placed as far back as possible without the horse taking a step forward. This removes the fetlock from the area of interest.
- The X-ray beam is directed proximal to distal 30° to 40°, depending on how far back the foot is placed.
- The beam is centred parallel to the long axis of the horse's leg and centred in the middle of the groove between the bulbs of the heel.
- Collimation should be limited to the area of the navicular bone (Figure 18.2).

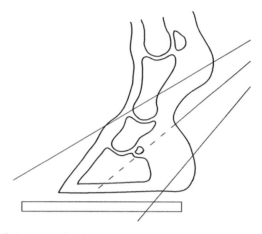

Figure 18.2 Palmaro-proximal–dorso-distal oblique of the navicular bone.

Fetlock

Dorso-palmar

- The horse should stand, bearing weight on all feet.
- The primary beam is angled down about 15° to ensure that it passes through the joint space.
- The film is placed in a film box behind the leg.
- The beam is centred on the articulation of the fetlock passing along the midline of the leg.
- Collimation should include the joint and a small area above and below the joint (Figure 18.3).

Latero-medial

- The horse should stand, bearing weight on all feet.
- The cassette is placed on the medial aspect of the leg and parallel to it.

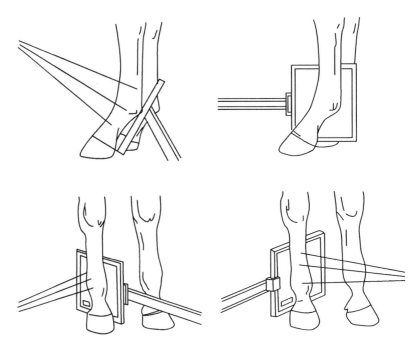

Figure 18.3   Positioning for the standard projections of the fetlock.

- The X-ray beam is centred on the articulation of the joint, parallel to the film.
- Collimation should include a small area above and below the joint.

Dorso-lateral–palmaro-medial oblique (D45L-PaMO) and dorso-medial–palmaro-lateral oblique (D45M-PaLO)

- The horse should stand, bearing weight on all four legs.
- The primary beam is directed perpendicular to the leg.
- For dorso-lateral–palmaro-medial oblique (DLPMO), the cassette is placed midway between the medial and palmar surfaces of the leg.
- For dorso-medial–palmaro-lateral oblique (DMPLO), the cassette is placed midway between the lateral and palmar surfaces of the leg. If the horse does not co-operate, then a plantar-lateral-dorso-medial oblique (PLDMO) is a safer projection to attempt as the X-ray tube and machine are not under the horse.
- The X-ray beam is centred on the articulation of the joint.

Metacarpus and metatarsus (cannon and splint)

Dorso-palmar

- The horse should stand, bearing weight on all feet.
- The film is placed in a film box or holder, behind the leg.
- The beam is centred on the middle of the cannon bone along the midline of the leg.
- Collimation should include the joints above and below the cannon bone.

Latero-medial

- The horse should stand, bearing weight on all feet.
- The cassette is placed on the medial aspect of the leg and parallel to it.
- The X-ray beam is centred on the centre of the cannon bone, parallel with the film.
- Collimation should include the joints above and below the cannon bone.

Dorso-lateral–palmaro-medial oblique (D45L-PaMO) and dorso-medial–palmaro-lateral oblique (D45M-PaLO)

- The horse should stand, bearing weight on all four legs.
- The primary beam is directed perpendicular to the leg.
- For DLPMO, the cassette is placed midway between the medial and palmar surfaces of the leg.
- For DMPLO, the cassette is placed midway between the lateral and palmar surfaces of the leg. If the horse does not co-operate, then a PLDMO is a safer projection to attempt as the X-ray tube and machine are not under the horse.
- The X-ray beam is centred on the centre of the cannon bone, parallel with the film.
- Collimation should include the joints above and below the cannon bone.
- If the splint bones are under examination, the oblique views should be taken with a reduced exposure (Figure 18.4).

Carpus

Dorso-palmar

- The horse should stand bearing weight on all feet.
- The film is placed in a film box or holder behind the leg.

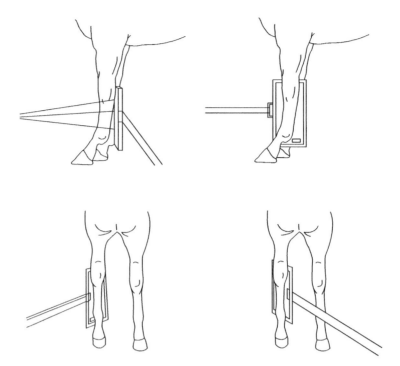

Figure 18.4   Positioning for the standard projections of the metacarpus or metatarsus.

- The beam is centred on the middle of the joint passing along the midline of the leg.
- Collimation should include the joint and a small area above and below.

Latero-medial

- The horse should stand, bearing weight on all feet.
- The cassette is placed on the medial aspect of the leg and parallel to it.
- The X-ray beam is centred on the middle of the joint, parallel with the film.
- Collimation should include a small area above and below the joint.

Dorso-lateral–palmaro-medial oblique (D45L-PaMO) and dorso-medial–palmaro-lateral oblique (D45M-PaLO)

- The horse should stand, bearing weight on all four legs.
- The primary beam is directed perpendicular to the leg.

- For DLPMO, the cassette is placed midway between the medial and palmar surfaces of the leg (Figure 18.5).
- For DMPLO, the cassette is placed midway between the lateral and palmar surfaces of the leg. If the horse does not co-operate, then a PLDMO is a safer projection to attempt as the X-ray tube and machine are not under the horse.
- The X-ray beam is centred on the middle of the joint.

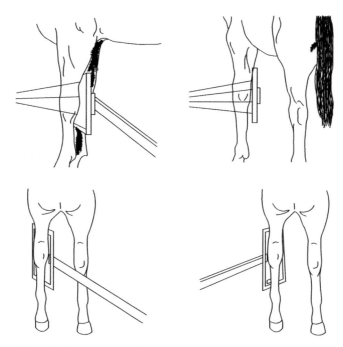

Figure 18.5 Positioning for standard projections of the carpus.

Elbow

Cranio-caudal

- The horse should stand, bearing weight on all legs.
- The limb under examination should be moved forward slightly to free it from the chest wall.
- The head should be turned away from the leg to free it from the chest wall.
- The cassette is angled and pushed up behind the elbow into the chest wall.
- In larger animals, a slight downward angulation may be necessary, or angulation of the beam from medial to lateral.

- The primary beam is centred on the distal margin of the humerus.
- Collimation should include a small amount of the radius and the humerus.

Lateral

- The film should be placed in a bucky or in a bag on a drip stand.
- The affected leg is placed next to the film with the horse standing.
- The leg under examination is then lifted forward and raised to reduce superimposition of the unaffected leg.
- The primary beam is centred on the joint, parallel with the film (Figure 18.6).
- The person lifting the limb should wear lead protection.

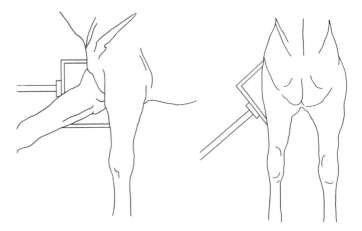

Figure 18.6   Positioning of the elbow.

Shoulder

Lateral

- The film should be placed in a bucky or in a bag on a drip stand.
- A grid should be used.
- The affected leg is placed next to the film with the horse standing.
- The leg under examination is then lifted forward and raised to reduce superimposition of the unaffected leg.
- Raising the leg will also place the trachea over the joint, which will improve the image quality.
- The primary beam is centred on the joint, parallel with the film (Figure 18.7).
- The person lifting the limb should wear lead protection.

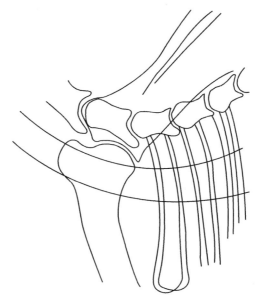

Figure 18.7   Positioning of the shoulder.

Tarsus

Dorso-palmar

- The horse should stand, bearing weight on all feet.
- The film is placed in a film box or holder behind the leg.
- The beam is centred on the middle of the joint passing along the midline of the leg.
- Collimation should include the joint and a small area above and below.

Latero-medial

- The horse should stand, bearing weight on all feet.
- The cassette is placed on the medial aspect of the leg and parallel to it.
- The X-ray beam is centred on the middle of the joint, parallel with the film.
- Collimation should include a small area above and below the joint.
- When imaging the hock, a slight angulation (10°) will improve image quality by allowing the primary beam to pass through the joint space.

Dorso-lateral–palmaro-medial oblique (D45L-PaMO) and
dorso-medial–palmaro-lateral oblique (D45M-PaLO)

- The horse should stand, bearing weight on all four legs.
- The primary beam is directed perpendicular to the leg.
- For DLPMO, the cassette is placed midway between the medial and palmar surfaces of the leg (Figure 18.8).

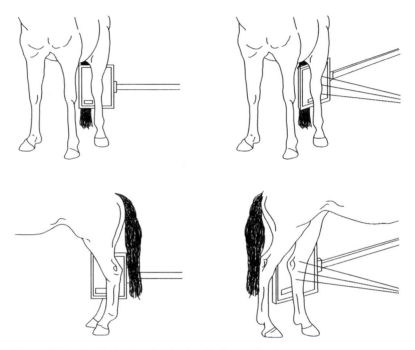

Figure 18.8   Positioning for standard projections of the tarsus.

- For DMPLO, the cassette is placed midway between the lateral and plantar surfaces of the leg. If the horse does not co-operate, then a PLDMO is a safer projection to attempt as the X-ray tube and machine are not under the horse.
- The X-ray beam is centred on the middle of the joint.

Stifle

Latero-medial

- The horse should have some contact around the stifle area before the examination begins.
- The horse should be bearing weight on all legs.

- A cassette is placed on the medial side of the horse's leg and rotated up as high as possible.
- This cassette is held and so adequate lead protection must be used.
- The long edge of the cassette should be visible on the cranial edge of the leg.
- The primary beam should be perpendicular to the cassette and the leg.
- The primary beam is centred at the base of the patella.
- The caudal aspect of the leg is not needed within the collimation as it only contains soft tissue.

Caudo-cranial

- The horse should have some contact around the stifle area before the examination begins.
- The horse should be bearing weight on all legs.
- A cassette is placed on the cranial side of the horse's leg and lifted as high as possible.
- This cassette is held and so adequate lead protection must be used.
- The long edge of the cassette should be visible on the lateral edge of the leg.
- The primary beam should be angled downwards about 10° so that it passes through the joint space.
- The primary beam is centred at the base of the patella (Figure 18.9).

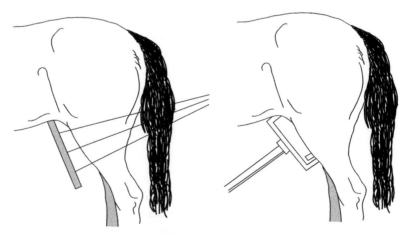

Figure 18.9   Positioning of the stifle.

Head

In the horse, imaging of the skull in the conscious patient is limited to a lateral projection. Further views can be taken under anaesthesia, but its details will not be given here.

Latero-medial skull and sinuses

- The film is placed in a bag hung on a drip stand.
- A grid is not needed.
- The horse stands with the affected side against the film holder.
- A rope head collar should be used to prevent artefacts from buckles and clips.
- The head is supported with a gloved hand.
- The primary beam is centred at the base of the facial crest perpendicular to the head and film (Figure 18.10).
- Collimation should include all of the maxilla, the frontal sinuses and the first cheek tooth.

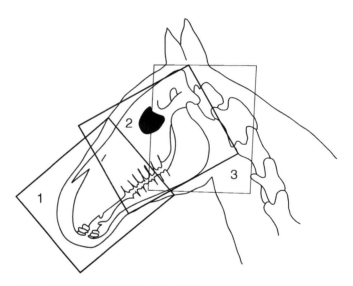

Figure 18.10   Positioning for the equine skull.

Spine

The spine of a horse can be easily imaged using a lateral projection with the horse standing. This is possible in general practice for the entire spine apart from the lumbar spine, beyond the diaphragm. The lumbar spine can be imaged, but there is increased scatter reducing the image quality, and a high mAs is essential.

The horse should stand parallel to the film. Positioning should be over the spine and include some overlap from film to film so that all articulations can be assessed. The thoracic spine should be radiographed in two separate parts: one for the vertebral bodies and one for the spinous processes (withers). A grid is essential for all images of the spine.

Chest

Imaging of the equine thorax needs to be carried out in four parts. The exposure factors should be increased for cranial images due to the increase in tissue density.

Collimation should be no bigger than the film used.

All projections are laterals.

If an image is to be diagnostic, either a grid or the air gap technique should be used (Figure 18.11).

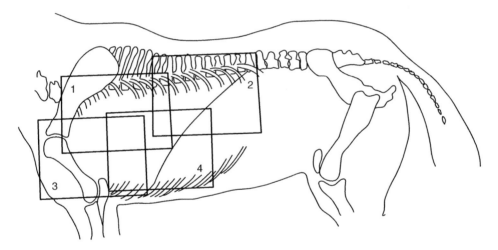

Figure 18.11   Arrangement of cassettes and centering for equine thorax.

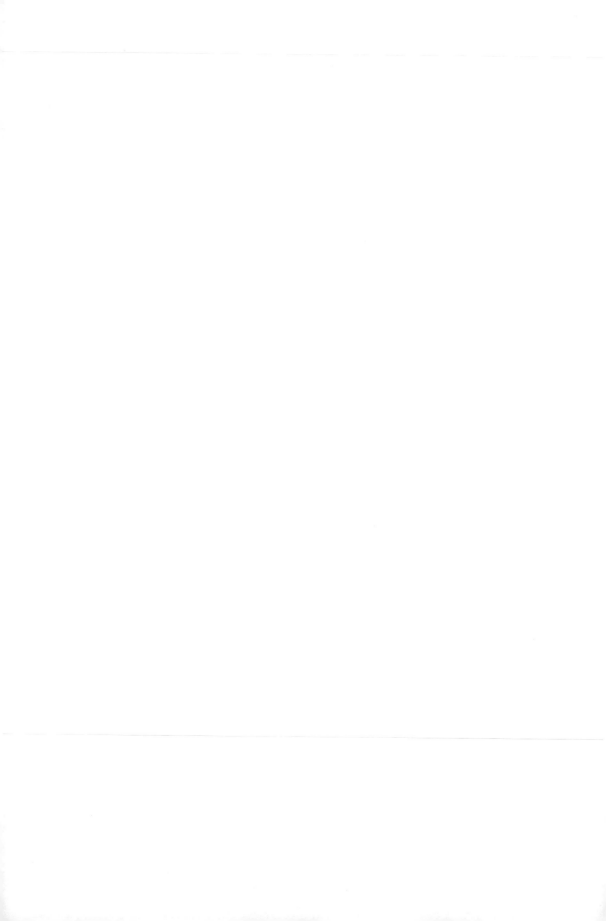

Chapter 19

Introduction to Ultrasound

Chapter contents

Sound waves
Ultrasound
How ultrasound works
Types of ultrasound scan
Doppler ultrasound
Effects on tissue
Ultrasound machines and transducers
Patient preparation
Areas suitable for examination
Further reading

Key points

- Ultrasound is high-frequency sound waves in the Megahertz (MHz) range
- Ultrasound is a form of non-ionising radiation
- Sound waves are created by the piezoelectric effect
- The sound waves are transmitted into the body and reflected back in varying amounts from an anatomical interface and these reflected waves are detected to produce an image
- Modern ultrasound machines contain a computer that generates the images and can send them either to film or a picture archiving communication system
- Ultrasound transducers have different frequencies and are usually in the range of 1–20 MHz
- The higher the frequency, the better the resolution, but poorer the penetration

Practical Veterinary Diagnostic Imaging, Second Edition. Suzanne Easton.
© 2012 John Wiley & Sons, Ltd. Published 2012 by Blackwell Publishing Ltd.

Introduction

Ultrasound was originally developed during World War I to track submarines as SONAR technology (SOund, Navigation And Ranging). Ultrasound was first used medically in the 1950s. It rapidly became available in the veterinary field and is now the second most utilised imaging technique. It does not expose the patient or operator to ionising radiation and there is minimal preparation required making it a quick and efficient diagnostic tool. It is, however, operator dependent and time should be taken to develop an understanding of the procedures to ensure a positive outcome for the patient.

Sound waves

Sound is a wave, which moves longitudinally. It is created by vibrating objects and moves via particle interaction from one location to another. Each particle pushes on its neighbouring particle and moves it in a forward direction. It then returns to its original position at the end of the interaction. This backward and forward movement is parallel to the direction of movement of the wave. In some areas of the wave, the particles are compressed together (compressions) and other areas the particles are spread apart (rarefactions).

The frequency of a wave refers to the number of complete back-and-forth vibrations (cycles) of a particle of the medium per unit of time. The hertz (Hz) is a unit for frequency where 1 Hz is equivalent to 1 cycle per second.

Ultrasound

Ultrasound is the use of very high frequency sound waves to produce a diagnostic image. These sound waves are above 10,000 Hz, which is well above the audible range of humans. Diagnostic ultrasound uses a range of 1–20 MHz.

How ultrasound works

Ultrasound is formed in waves from a transducer. The transducer consists of a ceramic crystal between two pincers. A current is applied to the pincers, which will pass through the crystal and crush it. When the voltage is applied to the ceramic, a pulse of high-frequency sound waves is produced. The sound wave will pass through the body and then bounce back, causing compression of the ceramic and the creation of an electrical impulse. This is known as piezo-electricity. This can be repeated a number of times a second as the process is very quick (Figure 19.1).

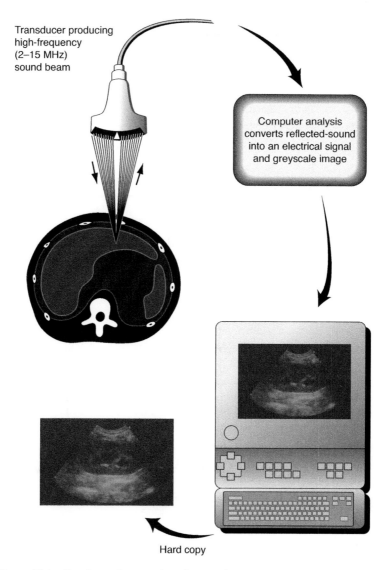

Transducer producing high-frequency (2–15 MHz) sound beam

Computer analysis converts reflected-sound into an electrical signal and greyscale image

Hard copy

Figure 19.1 Forming an image using ultrasound.

The speed of the ultrasound waves through soft tissues is 1540 m/s (Table 19.1). The impulses are amplified and displayed on a monitor to give a continuous image. These can then be frozen and printed or recorded on a video as a moving image (real time) to be viewed at a later date.

Different tissues have different resistance levels to the passage of sound and this will alter the reflection of the sound waves back to the transducer. This will alter the appearance of the tissues on the image produced and allows differentiation between tissue types.

Table 19.1 Speed of sound through various mediums.

Medium	Speed (m s^{-1})
Air	330
Water	1497
Fat	1440
Blood	1570
Metal	3000–6000
Soft tissue	1540

Types of ultrasound scan

A mode

This is the amplitude mode and the use of this is now limited. This uses a horizontal axis to show the depth into the patient of the tissue boundary and a vertical axis to show the strength of the echo. The larger the echo, the higher the peak (Figure 19.2).

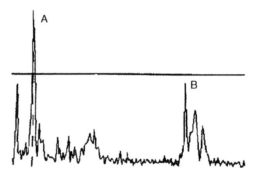

Figure 19.2 A mode ultrasound.

B mode

This is the brightness mode and is the most common mode in use today. Each reflecting echo registers as a bright spot, the larger the amplitude of the echo, the brighter the spot. The mode will use lots of scan lines from the source to produce a two-dimensional cross-section image. The image is changing all the time and allows the structures to be seen (Figure 19.3).

M mode

This is the movement mode and is used in cardiology as it allows the movement of structures to be shown as a frozen image (Figure 19.4).

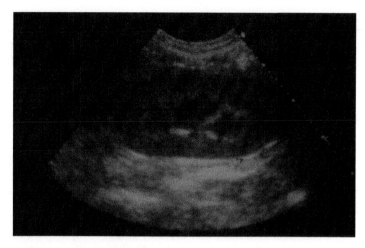

Figure 19.3   B mode ultrasound.

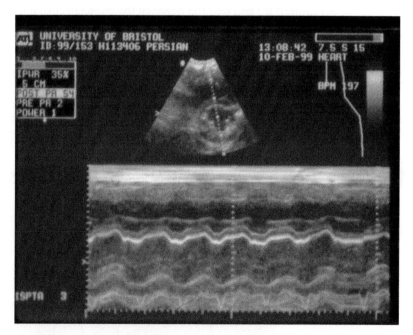

Figure 19.4   M mode ultrasound.

Doppler ultrasound

This technique uses the Doppler effect and is used to examine the movement of liquids. It can be used to demonstrate abnormalities in blood flow and to evaluate the flow through structures and also the velocity of the blood flow.

Effects on tissue

Ultrasound has not been shown to cause any long-term damage to tissue although research is still being carried out. It has, however, been shown to have some effect on tissues which do not cause long-term problems. Ultrasound will generate heat within the tissue and a micro-massaging effect. The combination of these two effects can be used in humans in a physiotherapy situation to benefit the patient. The ultrasound waves will also make all the electrons within the area of examination flow in the same direction and this effect is known as micro streaming.

Ultrasound machines and transducers

Ultrasound machines are now small, compact and incredibly mobile, making them easily stored and used even in a small practice. Wherever it is used, it is important to select a machine that is fit for the purpose it is required for and that the needs of the clinicians using the equipment and the patient types are taken into consideration during the selection process (Figure 19.5).

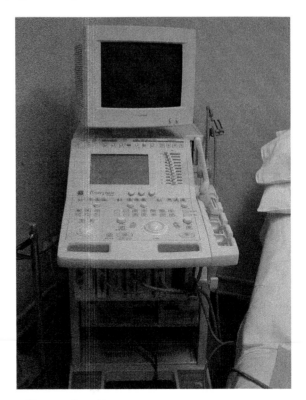

Figure 19.5 Ultrasound machine.

Transducers (also known as probes), come in a range of sizes and shapes, depending on the type of examination and the frequency required. The frequency also needs to be selected depending on the detail required and the size of the patient. A low-frequency transducer will image deep structures, but may not give a good-quality image when compared to a higher frequency probe (Figure 19.6).

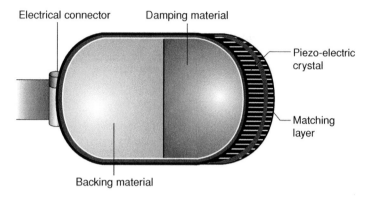

Figure 19.6 Ultrasound transducer.

Patient preparation

For the ultrasound examination to be effective, the animal must have the area prepared. This allows for the ultrasound waves to pass from the transducer into the patient and back again without interference from the air outside of the patient:

- The area for examination is clipped. Areas with underlying bone or gas should be avoided, as this will block the movement of the sound waves.
- Spirit is used to remove any residue dirt and grease on the skin surface.
- Coupling gel is applied to the transducer and the skin to ensure contact between the skin and transducer without the interference of air.

Areas suitable for examination

Ultrasound is becoming the examination of choice for the diagnosis of more and more diseases; however, it cannot replace all the tasks which radiography can perform. It is suitable for use in practices as it is mobile, easy to store and needs no specific precautions or areas for use. The main disadvantage is that operators need experience, and if this experience is lacking, diagnosis may be inaccurate.

The main areas of examination are abdominal soft tissue organs, the heart, thyroid, larynx, tendons, ligaments and soft tissue masses. It can also be used for pregnancy diagnosis, but is not accurate enough to determine numbers in small animals or sex.

Ultrasound can also be used as a means of guiding needles during biopsies, cystocentesis or fine needle aspirates.

Bone cannot be examined and may cause artefacts on the images of other regions if the ultrasound wave has to pass through or past bone to reach the area of interest. Large amounts of air can also obscure the area of interest and cause artefacts.

Further reading

McConnell, F. (2008) The use of ultrasonography in small animal veterinary practice. *Ultrasound* 16(3), 146–154.

Revision questions

1 How are sound waves generated?

2 What can Doppler ultrasound be used to demonstrate?

3 What is 'B mode' ultrasound?

4 How does coupling gel work?

5 Describe the patient preparation necessary for an ultrasound scan.

6 What is the piezo-electric effect?

7 Name two substances that ultrasound waves will not image accurately.

8 List three parts of the body that can be imaged using ultrasound.

9 What is a transducer?

10 What is the unit used to measure frequency?

Chapter 20

Advance Imaging Techniques

Chapter contents

Fluoroscopy
Computerised tomography (CT)
Magnetic resonance imaging (MRI)
Nuclear scintigraphy
Further reading

Key points

- Fluoroscopy provides an image that can be seen on a TV monitor as it happens (real time)
- The exposures required to produce a diagnostic image are very low
- Fluoroscopy can be used for barium swallow examinations, removal of foreign bodies or during interventional contrast examinations
- Computerised tomography provides cross-sectional cuts of the body
- CT uses ionising radiation and a detector
- CT can be used to demonstrate CNS disorders and tumours and gives more detail than conventional radiographic examinations
- MRI uses a large magnet with a radio frequency being applied to produce an image
- MRI is ideal for the demonstration of soft tissue structures including the spinal cord, joints and the brain
- Nuclear scintigraphy uses a radioisotope
- The isotope is injected into the animal, attached to a marker and will be taken to the organ or system of interest
- Scintigraphy is mainly used for examination of the bone and the thyroid tissue in small animals
- It can be used in equine examinations to detect bone defects not seen with conventional imaging

Practical Veterinary Diagnostic Imaging, Second Edition. Suzanne Easton.
© 2012 John Wiley & Sons, Ltd. Published 2012 by Blackwell Publishing Ltd.

Introduction

In veterinary practice, the imaging modalities available are limited, but an understanding of all the available possibilities and how these would benefit a patient are essential. Conventional radiography can be expanded to include fluoroscopy. Computerised tomography and magnetic resonance imaging are becoming more available to practices as more freelance imaging services become available. An understanding of the possibilities and the limitations of magnetic resonance imaging, computerised tomography and nuclear scintigraphy will benefit the care and treatment of a patient.

Fluoroscopy

The fluoroscopy unit uses a basic X-ray tube attached to an image intensifier. This converts the X-rays emerging from the patient into light and then multiplies the intensity of this light and converts it to photoelectrons through the use of a photocathode. The photocathode directs the electrons towards the output phosphor and an anode. The photoelectrons arriving at the output phosphor are 50 to 70 times brighter. This reduces the dose, which is necessary to produce a suitable image. The photoelectrons are then used to form a television or digital image that can be viewed. The quality of the image obtained is only as good as the monitor displaying the image. The size of the focal spot can be altered to magnify the image and enhance viewing further (Figure 20.1).

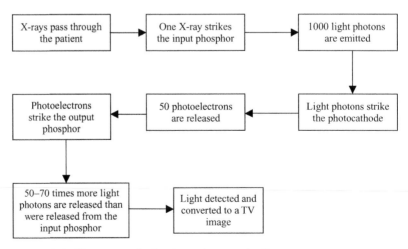

Figure 20.1   The process for forming an image using fluoroscopy.

The image displayed on the monitor will appear as the reverse of a conventional radiograph. Bone will be shown as black, the lungs will appear as white. The image produced using fluoroscopy, gives a moving image that can be recorded on video or it can be stored on 10 cm × 10 cm film in the normal way. These films are exposed using a very short exposure time so that multiple exposures can be made. On machines available to veterinary practice, up to 3 frames a second are possible. The images produced will be 'normal radiographs' with bone appearing white and lungs will be black. When setting up a fluoroscopy unit, the image intensifier should be as close to the patient as possible, preferably above the patient (Figure 20.2).

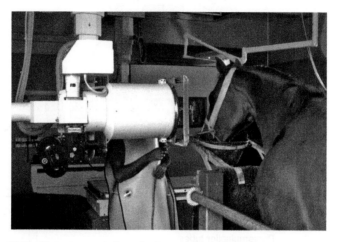

Figure 20.2   Fluoroscopy during a barium swallow of a horse.

Uses of fluoroscopy

Fluoroscopy can be used anytime that a real-time (moving) image is needed. This includes barium swallow examinations, the removal of oesophageal foreign bodies and some interventional procedures such as angiography or portosystemic shunts. It can also be used during orthopaedic surgery to check the position of screws, but care must be taken with radiation safety when using it in this situation.

Problems with fluoroscopy

The problems encountered with fluoroscopy are the same as those for general radiography including suitable sedation and positioning. There is, however, less of a problem with the dose received by staff and patients as the exposure is minimal. This does not mean that safety precautions can be relaxed. Lead aprons must be worn at all times when fluoroscopy is being used.

Computerised tomography (CT)

This technique produces images of selected thin cross-sectional slices of the body. Conventional radiography produces images that are parallel to the long axis of the body; CT produces a transverse image (an image that appears to have sliced the patient from front to back and from head to tail in sequence; Figure 20.3).

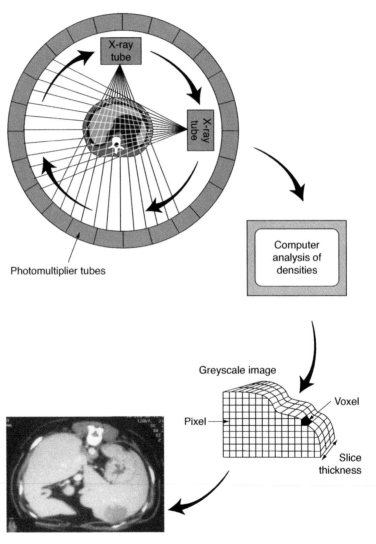

Figure 20.3   Principles of CT scanning.

How it works

A scout image is produced. This demonstrates the whole body and from this the areas for examination can be determined. The patient is examined from lots of angles by a thin X-ray beam using the principles of tomography. The X-ray tube and detector will move around the patient at one level and then the examination table will advance the patient through the scanner so a further slice at the next level can be acquired (Figure 20.4). At this stage, no image is actually formed. The radiation that has passed through the patient is picked up by a detector and fed into a computer. This data is recorded as a series of numbers and is then reconstructed into a digital image by the computer and displayed on a monitor. This can then be manipulated to produce a diagnostic image. The images can then be stored on a disk or on normal X-ray type film. The image is in the form of lots of small units called pixels. Each pixel has a numerical value known as a CT number. They are measured in Hounsfield units. Water has a Hounsfield unit of zero, air -1000 and muscle 50. All tissue types within the body will have different Hounsfield units.

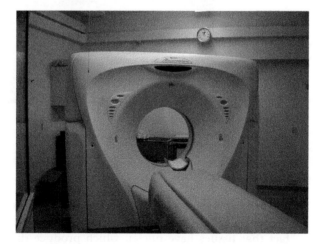

Figure 20.4   CT scanner.

Problems with CT

The only problems with this type of examination are:

1 The patient must remain still for the whole examination. Patient movement will result in a blurred image and inaccurate slices. Between slices, the table will move the patient further through the

scanner. This may cause movement if the patient is not adequately restrained using anaesthesia.

2 The usual safety considerations during the use of ionising radiation need to be followed. This includes ensuring that only necessary people are in the room during exposures. Due to the nature of the examination, this is usually for the entire acquisition period.

Uses

CT is useful in the diagnosis and staging of tumours and the diagnosis of central nervous system disorders. It can also be used to supplement any radiological examination where more detail is needed (Figure 20.5).

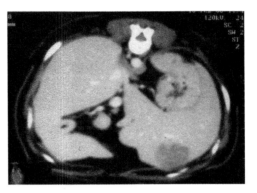

Figure 20.5   CT image of an abdomen.

Magnetic resonance imaging (MRI)

MRI uses a magnetic field and the effect a certain radio frequency has on this field to produce a radio signal. This effect relies on the fact that tissues have nuclei, which produce different radio signals, dependent on their atomic number. When the patient is in the scanner, a magnetic field is applied around their body. This makes all the atoms spin. A radio signal is then applied to the area and this makes the atoms relax back to their original position. The time it takes for this relaxation to occur depends on the atomic number of the nucleus. Different materials relax at a different speeds and this determines the density on the image, which is produced by the computer system. The big advantage of MRI is that it does not use ionising radiation (Figure 20.6).

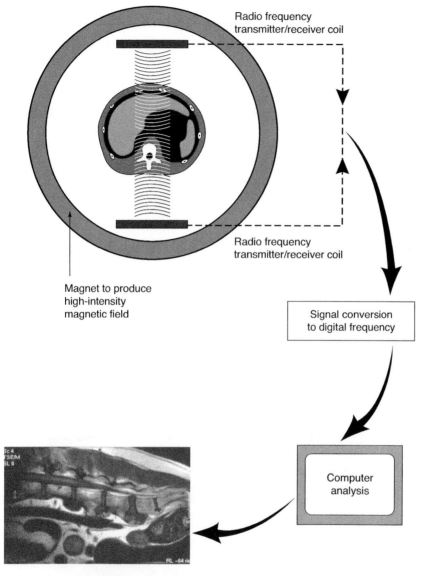

Figure 20.6   Principles of MRI scanning.

Problems with MRI

Due to the presence of the magnetic field and radio signal, a number
of precautions need to be taken:

- Patients with pacemakers or a new prosthesis must not enter the
  scanner room.

- Credit cards and anything with a magnetic strip will be wiped if they are taken into the scanner room.
- Metal objects should not be taken into the scanner room, as they will move very quickly towards the bore of the magnet. This includes scalpels, needles, oxygen cylinders or trolleys.
- A coil must be placed around the area under examination. This looks like a tube, but actually plays a vital role in applying the radio frequency.
- The scanner can be noisy.
- Examination times can be long and so anaesthesia is necessary to reduce patient movement.

Areas suitable for examination

MRI is more sensitive than CT for investigation of the nervous system. This includes the brain and the associated blood and nerve supply. MRI will also demonstrate spinal cord lesions very well. MRI has very poor definition for bone and structures containing calcium, but is very good for associated muscle and joint composition. The technique is also very good for showing abnormalities in the thorax including tumours and vascular anomalies. Contrast agents can be used to enhance the image if it is thought to have a blood supply (Figure 20.7).

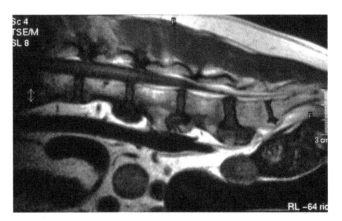

Figure 20.7   MRI image of the lumbar spine.

Nuclear scintigraphy

This type of examination uses a radioactive isotope attached to a compound that will be taken up by a certain substance in the body (e.g.

bone, thyroid tissue) following injection into the circulatory system. After a set period of time, the patient is placed in front of a detector and the amount of radiation emitted from certain points is recorded and evaluated against the expected normal values. In an area where there is an abnormality, the isotope will either be present in a higher amount (hot spot) or not present at all (cold spot). The uptake can either be recorded on a hand-held probe giving counts at certain points or on a gamma camera, which will show the images on a monitor (Figure 20.8).

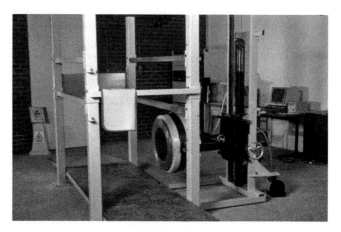

Figure 20.8 Gamma camera ready for an equine examination.

The gamma camera

The gamma camera is the most accurate method of detecting the gamma radiation emitted by the patient. The camera consists of a large sodium iodide crystal. This will convert the gamma radiation to light. Photomultiplier tubes convert the light into electrical pulses, then detect the light. The photomultiplier tubes amplify these electrical pulses. The electrical pulses are counted by an electronic monitor and plotted on a television monitor to give a diagnostic image.

The front of the gamma camera has a collimator that acts in a similar way to a grid. It will remove all low-energy gamma radiation and any radiation that is not moving in a forward direction. This will improve the quality of the resultant image (Figure 20.9).

Radiopharmaceuticals used

Radioisotopes are used in scintigraphy to provide the gamma radiation for detection. The isotopes are usually attached to a marker,

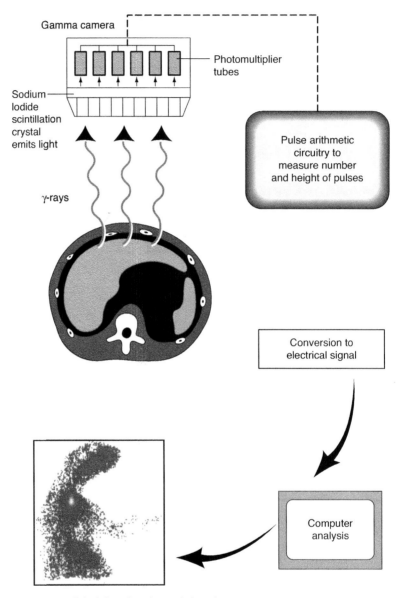

Figure 20.9 Principles of nuclear scintigraphy.

depending on the organ to be examined. The most commonly used isotope in the veterinary field is technetium-99m. The technetium has a half-life of 6 hours and an energy level of 140 keV, making it ideal for veterinary use.

Technetium can be attached to various compounds to allow it to target certain organs or body systems.

Hydroxymethylene diphosphonate (HDP) will target bone; thyroid tissue as well as the stomach and the salivary glands will take up technetium pertechnetate (Figure 20.10).

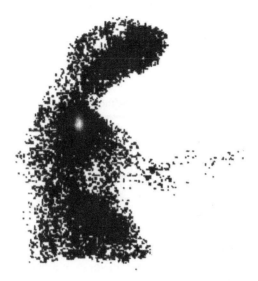

Figure 20.10   Thyroid scan of a cat with hyperthyroidism.

Problems with scintigraphy

There are two major problems when using scintigraphy:

1 The patients need to be isolated for a minimum of 48 hours after the isotope has been injected before it reaches a safe level. This means that the animal must be isolated for this period and that all their waste must be stored for the same period of time before it can be disposed of.
2 The patient must be kept very still while the scan is performed. If they move, the counts will produce a false image and this may lead to a misdiagnosis. Sedation must be good, but the animals must not wobble or sway if they are standing for the scan.

Regions suitable for investigation

Scintigraphy can be used to demonstrate bone in all animals. This will show stress fractures, tumours or other bony pathology. In cats, it can be used to show the thyroid position and size. This is of diagnostic use because normal thyroid tissue will take up the radiopharmaceutical in similar amounts as the parotid salivary gland. If the thyroid is over active, this uptake will increase and the thyroid tissue will appear 'hotter' than the salivary gland. It can also be used to show kidneys, lungs and abdominal organs, but this use is limited in the veterinary field. Scintigraphy is also used in cases with suspected porto-systemic shunts to determine the fraction of blood bypassing the liver.

Further reading

Avner, A. (2010) Computed tomographic imaging of migrating inhaled foreign plant material and its sequelae. *Companion Animal* 15(7), 81–86.

Mannion, P. (2009) CT of the thorax. *Companion Animal* 14(9), 42–46.

All of the techniques in this chapter are becoming more available to veterinary practice. If a patient is referred for examination, take time to follow up the case and view the images.

Revision questions

1 Describe how an image intensifier works.

2 Give three situations where fluoroscopy would be of use.

3 If you were using digital imaging, what would you not have to use?

4 Does CT produce transverse or longitudinal images?

5 Describe how atoms move during an MRI scan.

6 What must you not take into an MRI scanner room?

7 What are the parts that make up a gamma camera?

8 How does the radioisotope reach the structure of interest?

9 List two structures that can be imaged using nuclear scintigraphy.

Index

Note: Page number(s) with italicised *f*'s and *t*'s refer to figures and tables, respectively.

abdomen, positioning, 191–2
absorbed dose, 6
absorption, 75
  photoelectric, 72–3, 53
accelerator, 111
acidifier, 113
actinic marker, 166
active matrix array (AMA), 131
air, 172
air-gap technique, 86–7
ALARA principle, 154
alkali metals, 28
alkali solution, 111
ammonium thiosulphate, 112
amorphous selenium detector, 132
amorphous silicon detector, 131
amperes (amps), 4
angiography, 186
animal radiography, terminology with, 167
anode, 40–41
  heel effect, 45
  stationary anodes, 43
anode-heel effect, 45, 145
anti-halation layer, 92–3
  effect, 93
  film 90, 93
anti-scatter grid, 82
anti-sludging agent, 113–14
arthrography, 184–6
atom
  make-up of, 27
  nucleus, 19
  shell, 22, 28
  structure, 27
atomic number, 29, 142
  attenuation, 78, 105
  diaphragm, 161, 190
atomic shells, electrons, 28
attenuation, 75
automatic processor
  care of, 115
  dryer systems, 115–16
  film transport system, 114–15
  water systems and drainage, 114–15

badge, film, 158
bandages, 165
barium enema, 177–8
barium sulphate, 172–3, 176, 187
barium swallow, 175
bar magnet, magnetic fields in, 19. *See also* magnet
base of screen, 101
base units, 4
beam-centring devices, 81
beam filtration, 38–9
becquerel (Bq), 7, 9
benzotriazole, 111
birds, 103–4, 203–4
boric acid, 113
braking radiation, 63
bremsstrahlung X-ray spectrum, 65
  characteristics, 65
bremsstrahlung radiation, 63, 70
  production, 63
British Veterinary Association, 168–9
bromine atoms, 94
buffer, 113

caesium iodide (CsI), 131
calcium tungstate, 101, 103
carbon, 29
carpus, 209–10
  positioning, 211
cathode, 40
caudo-cranial shoulder, 210
ceilings of darkroom, 119
cells, radiation damage, 154
characteristic curve, 139–40
  shoulder, 140
  straight-line portion, 140
  toe, 139
characteristic radiation, 64
charts, exposure, 70
chemical fogging, 111
chest radiography, 189–91
circuit breaker, 56
cisternal puncture, 183
classical scattering, 72
coating, protective, 100

collimation, 205
compression band, 81
Compton effect, 72, 74
Compton scatter, 74
computed radiography, *see also* digital radiography
    computerised process, 129–30
    erasure of plate, 128
    imaging plate, 127–8
    imaging plate and cassette, care of, 129
    latent image, retrieval of, 128–9
computerised tomography, 230–32
    uses, 232
conduction, definitions of, 3*t*
conductors, 14
    radiation dose, 75
contrast, 141–4
    examination procedures, 175–82
        angiography, 186
        arthrography, 184, 185*f*
        dacryocystorhinogram, 186
        fistulography, 185
        portal venography, 185
        sinography, 185
        venography, 186
    film contrast, 143
    film fogging, 143
    kilovoltage, 143
    media, 144
        myelography, 182–4
        negative, 172
        positive, 172–5, 173*t*
    object shape and thickness, 143
control panel, 54
controlled area, 156–7
convection, definitions of, 3
COSHH regulations, 121
coulombs (Q), 7, 13
CR, *see* computed radiography
cross-hatched parallel grid, 85
current, types of, 15–16
cystography, 181–2

dacryocystorhinogram, 186
darkroom, 118–21
    doors, 119
    floors, 119
    safelights, 120–21
    size, 119
    ventilation, 119
    walls and ceilings, 119
    white lights, 119–20
densitometry, 138
density
    of film, 141
    tissue, 143
developer
    accelerator, 111
    developing agents, 111
    fungicide, 112
    hardener, 112
    preservative, 111
    restrainer, 111
    sequestering agents, 111
    solvent, 112
developing agents, 111
development of film, 108–9

diaphragm box, 80
digital imaging, *see also* computed radiography;
        digital radiography
    chart, 126*f*
    overview of, 125–7
digital mobile X-ray unit, 58
digital radiography, *see also* computed radiography
    direct, 132–3, 132*f*
    image display, 134
    image quality, 135
    image storage, 133
    indirect, 131–2
dipoles, 21
direct digital radiography, 132–3
direct safelights, 121
disintegration, definition of, 7
distal extremities, 196–9
distortion, 144–6
dorsal-ventral chest radiography, 190
dorso-lateral–palmaro-medial oblique
        (D45L-PaMO), 208
dose area product (DAP) meter, 54
dose limits, 157–8
double contrast cystography, 182
DP projection, 206
drainage, water systems and, 114–15
dressings, 69–70
dryer systems, 115–16
drying film, 110–11
dual-focus tubes, 40–41
duplitised film, 94
dynamo, usage of, 22. *See also* electromagnetism

elbow, 211–12
    positioning, 199, 212
    scoring scheme, 168–9
electromagnetic radiation (EMR), 30–31
electromagnetic spectrum, 32
electrons, trapped, 128
emission spectrum, effect of mA, 66
EMR spectrum, 31
emulsion, 91–2
emulsion film
    duplitised, 90
    single-sided, 90
erasure of plate, 128
ethylene-diamine-tetra-acetic acid (EDTA),
        111
examination procedures (contrast), 175–82
excitation, 30–31
exposure charts, 70
electrical circuits, components of, 18
electric charge, 13
    measurement of, 13
electric current, laws of, 16
electricity, 14
    measuring, 14–15
electromagnetic induction, laws of
    Faraday's law, 22
    Fleming's left hand rule, 22
    Lenz's law, 22
electromagnetism, 20–22
    definition of, 21
electromotive force, 13, 15
electron
    ionisation effects, 31

electron spin, 19
electrostatics, 12–13
    creation of, 12–13
emission spectrum, 66
    atomic number effect, 66
    filtration effect, 67
    mA, effect, 66
energy, 2–3
    conversion, 2–3
    definition of, 2
    types of, 2t
exposure, 102, 127, 130
    radiation, 139
exposure devices, automatic, 56

Faraday's law, 22
ferromagnetism, 20
fetlock, 207–8
    positioning, 208
FFD, 70
filament circuit, 54
film
    badge, 158, 158f
    care and storage, 95–6
    contrast, 143
    density of, 141
    drying of, 110–11
    faults, 147–52
    fixing, 109–10
    fogging, 143
    hangers, 151
    screen film, 93
    selection, 101–2
    transport system, 114–15
    washing, 110
film base, 91
film-object distance, 144
film-screen combinations, 101–4, see also intensifying
        screens
film sensitivity, 96–7
    assessment, 97
    calculation, 97
filtration, effect, 67
fistulography, 185
fixer, 117
    acidifier, 113
    anti-sludging agent, 113–14
    buffer, 113
    fixing agent, 112
    hardener, 113
    preservative, 113
    solvent, 113
fixing agent, 112
fixing film, 109–10
Fleming's left hand rule, 22
floppy sandbags, 165
fluorescence, 77
fluorescent phosphor layer, 101
fluoroscopy, 228–9
focal film distance (FFD), 68
focal object distance (FOD), 144
focussing cup, 40
    function, 42
focus-to-grid distance, 84
football pitch, 27
frequency (ν), 33

frontal sinuses, 194
fungicide, 112

gap fills, 73
gastrointestinal tract, 175–8
genito-urinary tract, 178–82
gerbils, 202–3
gelatine, 91
generators
    electrical energy, 51
    high-voltage, 51
globular grains, 91–2
gray (Gy), 6
grid, 69
    construction, 82
    effect, 83
    factor, 83
    function, 81
    lattice, 83
    ratio, 82–3
    types, 84
    use, 69
guinea pigs, 202

hamsters, 202–3
hardener, 112–13
hardware artifacts, 135
head and neck radiography, see small animal
        radiography techniques
heat, definition of, 3
high-speed projectile electrons, 63
high-tension circuit, 55
high-voltage generators, 51
hip dysplasia, 168–9
hobbles, 165
hoof wall, 206
horizontal automatic processors, 116

image
    blur, 101
    display, 134
    quality, 145
        hardware artefacts, 135
        object artefacts, 135
        software artefacts, 135
image degradation, 74
imaging plate, construction of, 127
indirect digital radiography (IDR), 131–2
indirect safelighting, 121
intensifying screens
    care of, 104–5
    characteristics of, 100
    construction of, 100–101
        base, 101
        fluorescent phosphor layer, 101
        protective coating, 100
        reflective layer, 100–101
    cross-sectional view of, 100
    film-screen combinations
        light emission and film selection,
            101–2
        quantum mottle, 104
        single-screen use, 103
        speed, 102
        speed assessment, 103
    film-screen contact, 104

International System of Units (SI), 4
    base units, 4
    units in radiography, 5
inverse square law, 8–9
ionising radiation
    on body, 154
    regulations, 1999, 155
ionising radiation effects, types, 77
ionisation, effects, 31
interactions, characteristic, 64
interlocks, 56
intravenous urography, 178–9
iodine compounds, 173–5
    isotopes, 29–30

joules (J), 2

kilovoltage, 81, 143
kilovolts (kV), 4
kilowatts (kW), 3
kV, 69
kV compensator, 53
kVp, 66

labelling of radiographs, 166
laminitis, 206
laparotomy, 185
latitude, film, 140
laws, of electric current, 16
laws of electromagnetic induction
    Faraday's law, 22
    Fleming's left hand rule, 22
    Lenz's law, 22
lead shielding, 159–60, 160f
legends, 165–6
Lenz's law, 22
light beam diaphragm, 80
light-beam diaphragm checks, 161
light emission and film selection, 101–2
light-tight drawer, 96
low-energy photons, 67
lumbar puncture, 183
lumbar sacral junction, 201
luminescence, 77

macro-radiography, 144
magnet
    function and composition of, 19
    types of, 20
magnetic flux, 21
magnetic induction, 21
magnetic laws, 20
    attraction and repulsion, 20
    pairs, existence of poles in, 20
magnetic resonance imaging, 20, 232–4
magnetism, 17
    definition of, 17
magnification, 144–5
male retrograde urethrogram, 180
mammals
    images, 203
    rabbits and guinea pigs, 202
    small, 202
matter, 1
    definition of, 1

metacarpus and metatarsus (cannon and splint),
        209
mice, 202–3
milliamperes (mA), 4, 6
mobile units, 58
monitoring devices
    film bandage, 158
    thermoluminescent dosimeter, 159
movement and image quality, 145
myelography, 182–4, 184f

nasal chambers, 194–5
nasopharynx, 196
navicular bone, 205
negative contrast medium, 172
neutrons, 27
noise on image, 132
non-screen film, 94
nucleon or mass number, 29
    palmaro-proximal–dorso-distal oblique of,
        207

object artefacts, 135
object shape and thickness, 143
Ohm's law, 16
oil, 37
open film badge, 158f
orthochromatic film, 97
orthochromatic lights, 91
outline of, 107–8

parallel grid, 84
peak sensitivity, 97
pedal bone (DPr60°-PaDiO), 205
pelvis, positioning, 200–201, 210
penumbra, 44–5
periodic table, 28–9
phosphors, 101, 131
photoelectric absorption, 72–3
photoelectric absorption process, 73
photographic density, 141
photomultiplier, 128
photostimulable phosphors (PSP), 127–8, 127f
picture archiving and communications system
        (PACS), 133, 133f
Planck's constant, 33
pneumocystogram, 182f
polaroid imaging, 122
portal venography, 185
positioning aids, 165
positive contrast cystography, 182
positive contrast medium
    barium sulphate, 172–3, 173t
    iodine compounds, 173–5, 174t
    polyester, 91
power, 3
    definition of, 3
    measurement of, 3
preservative, 111, 113
processor, 161
proportions, 7
protective coating, 100
protons, 27, 29
psuedo-focussed grid, 84–5
Pyrex glass envelope, 37

quality assurance (QA)
 light-beam diaphragm checks, 161
 processor, 161
 X-ray machine, 160
quantum mottle, 104

rabbits, 202
radiation
 definitions of, 3
 effects on body, 154
 monitoring film, 94
 protection
  areas around X-ray machine, 156–7
  dose limits, 157–8
  ionising radiation on body, 154
  ionising radiation regulations 1999,
   155
  lead shielding, 159–60, 160*f*
  monitoring devices, 158–9, 159*f*
  overview of, 153–4
  quality assurance (QA), 160–61
  in veterinary practice, 155–6
 safety in veterinary practice
  local rules, 155–6
  system of work, 156

radiation protection advisor (RPA), 155–6
radiation protection supervisor (RPS),
  155–6
radioactivity, 30
radiographic film, 100
 construction, 90
radiographic film processing
 automatic processor, 114–15, 115–16*f*
 COSHH regulations, 121
 darkroom, 118–21, 118*f*
 polaroid, 122
 replenishment, 116–17
 silver recovery, 117–18
 stages of, 108–13, 109*f*
  developer, 111–12
  development, 108–9
  drying, 110–11
  fixer, 112–13
  fixing, 109–10
  washing, 110
 thermal imaging, 122
 video, 122
radiographic image quality
 characteristic curve, 139–40, 139*f*
 contrast, 141–4, 142*f*
 densitometry, 138
 density, 141, 141*f*, 141*t*
 distortion, 144–5, 146*f*
 film faults, 147–52
 high-quality of, 146
 latitude, 140, 140*f*
 magnification, 144, 145*f*
 movement, 145
 sensitometry, 138
radiography
 application of laws in, 23
 assessment of, 166
 BVA/KC hip dysplasia and elbow scoring scheme,
  168–9

markers and legends, 165–6
positioning aids, 165
principles, 164
restraint, 164
SI units in, 5*t*
terminology, 166–8, 167*f*, 168*t*
units and prefixes in, 3–4
 SI base units, 4
 standard scientific notation, 4, 4*t*
radiological units, 4–5, 5*t*
 absorbed dose, 6
 activity, 7
 dose equivalent, 6–7
 exposure in air, 7
 heat units, 6
 keV, 6
 kVp, 5–6
 mA/mAs, 6
radiolucent foam, 165
rectification, 51–2
reflective layer, 100–101
replenishment
 in automatic processor, 117
 during manual processing, 116–17
 starter solution and mixing chemicals, 117
reptiles, 204
resistance, 16
restrainer, 111
restraint, 145, 164, 190
rhenium, 43–4
roller system from processor, 115

safelights, 120–1, 120*f*
 direct, 121, 121*f*
 indirect, 121, 121*f*
 on light transmission, 130*f*
scatter, 132
 radiation, 159
scattered radiation, 81
scintigraphy, 234–6
screen, *see also* intensifying screens
 cleaning of, 104–5
 intensifying
  care of, 104–5
  construction of, 100–101
  view of, 100*f*
 single, 103
 speed of, 102
 speeds, 102*t*
secondary radiation, 81
sensitometry, 138
sequestering agents, 111
shells and energy, 28
shoulder
 arthrogram, 185
 positioning, 199
 radiography, 198–200
silver atoms, 94–5
silver halide, 95
 crystals, 109
 reaction, 95
silver halide crystal, 94
silver halide grains, 91
silver recovery, 117–18
sinography, 185

skull
  box, 165
  lateral, 193, 194*f*
  lateral oblique, 196
  ventro-dorsal, 192–3, 193*f*
small animal radiography techniques
  abdomen
    right lateral recumbency, 191–2, 192*f*
    ventro-dorsal (VD), 192
  birds
    lateral, 203, 204*f*
    ventro-dorsal, 203
  chest
    dorsal–ventral (DV), 190, 190*f*
    right lateral recumbency, 189, 190*f*
    ventro-dorsal (VD), 191, 191*f*
  distal extremities
    caudo-cranial, 197–8, 198–9*f*
    medio-lateral, 196–7, 197*f*
  head and neck
    dorso-ventral intra-oral view, 194, 195*f*
    lateral oblique skull, 196
    lateral skull, 193, 194*f*
    nasopharynx, 196
    oblique projection of teeth, 196
    open mouth rostro-caudal view, 194, 195*f*
    rostro-caudal view, 194
    ventro-dorsal skull, 192–3, 193*f*
  mammals, 202–3, 203*f*
  pelvis
    lateral, 200–201
    ventro-dorsal, 200, 201*f*
  reptiles, 204
  shoulder
    caudo-cranial, 200, 200*f*
    lateral, 198, 199*f*
  spine
    lateral, 201–2
    lumbar sacral junction (lateral), 201
    ventro-dorsal, 202
SMPTE test pattern, 134
sodium salt, 111
software artifacts, 135
solenoid, 20
solvent, 112–13
SONAR technology, 220
sound waves, 220
source–image distance (SID), 56, 68
space charge compensator, 55
spinal pain, 184
spine
  positioning, 201–2
standard scientific notation, 4. *See also* radiography
starter solution, 117
stationary anodes, 43
step wedge, 138
supervised area, 157
supply switch, 52

tabular grains, 92
teeth
  oblique projection of, 196
temperature, 3
temporo-mandibular joints (TMJ), 196
tesla (T), 21
thermal circuit breaker, 56

thermal imaging, 122
thermoluminescent dosimeter, 159, 159*f*
thin-filmtransistor (TFT), 132
thoracic myelogram, 184
timers, 55
tissue density and atomic number, 143
torch beam, usage of, 9
total energy, 2
trapped electrons, 128
tube port, 39
tube rating, 46–7
tympanic bullae, 194, 196

urethrogram
  female, 180–81
  male, 179–80
ultrasound, 219–20, 224
  types, 222

venography, 186
ventilation of darkroom, 119
ventro-dorsal chest radiography, 191–2
vertical automatic processors, 116
video imaging, 122
voltmeter, 53
volts, 14

walls of darkroom, 119
washing film, 110
water-soluble iodine compounds, 173–5, 174*t*
watts (W), 15
wavelength (λ), 32–3
wetting agent, 112
white lights, 119–20

X-ray beam, 74–5, 93, 208
X-ray circuit, 50–51
X-ray emission spectrum, 64
  characteristic radiation, 64
X-ray equipment, 96
X-ray exposures, 73
X-ray film, 96
  emulsion, 109
X-ray image, 73
X-ray interactions, 29
X-ray machine, 53
  areas around
    controlled area, 156–7
    supervised area, 157
  quality assurance, 160
X-ray machines
  fixed, 57–8
  power rating, 59
  types, 56
X-ray photons, 31, 33, 72, 74, 77
X-ray quality, 68
X-ray quantity, 68
X-ray tube, 2
  port, 38
  schematic diagram, 36
X-rays, 71
  production, 62
X-ray units, 57
  mobile, 58
  portable, 58
X-Rite tape, 166

Printed and bound by CPI Group (UK) Ltd, Croydon, CR0 4YY

27/10/2024

14580289-0001